NO FILTERS

No Filters

A Mother–Teenage Daughter Love Story

CHRISTIE WATSON AND ROWAN EGBERONGBE

Chatto & Windus

LONDON

1 3 5 7 9 10 8 6 4 2

Chatto & Windus, an imprint of Vintage, is part of the Penguin Random House group of companies whose addresses can be found at global.penguinrandomhouse.com

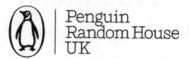

First published in the UK by Chatto & Windus in 2025

penguin.co.uk/vintage

Printed and bound in Great Britain by Clays Ltd, Elcograf S.p.A.

The authorised representative in the EEA is Penguin Random House Ireland, Morrison Chambers, 32 Nassau Street, Dublin DO2 YH68

A CIP catalogue record for this book is available from the British Library

ISBN 9781784744595

Penguin Random House is committed to a sustainable future for our business, our readers and our planet. This book is made from Forest Stewardship Council® certified paper.

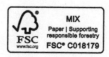

Gen Z × Gen X is an equation even Einstein would have struggled with.

For every teenager who is living through this time of times, and every parent who is trying to keep them safe.

Trigger Warning: Discussions on mental illness, suicide, racism, transphobia, self-harm, and eating disorders.

Contents

Authors' Note

This book is based on real events. However, names and details have been changed in order to protect identities. Kai, for example, is made up of composite experiences.

We would like readers to know that even with two sensitivity reads, legal advice and a brilliant editorial team all checking tone as well as words, there may be some content, or language, that will be triggering for some people. We are sorry if we have caused anyone offence. We wrote this book together, each working on own sections, checking each other's, and carefully editing. Both of us have done our best to write our truth and represent our individual experiences in a sensitive way, whilst acknowledging that our story will be completely different from other people's. This includes the language used. We both chose to use she/her pronouns and gendered words in this book, such as 'daughter'. Other people might prefer to use other language for themselves. The process of living through the last few years as well as writing together had us changing our minds about many difficult subjects. We will – no doubt – change our minds about many things in the future. There are millions of parents and teens out there, all figuring out how to navigate in their own unique and individual and complex and messy and beautiful ways. *No Filters* is our story.

Introduction

The teenage years can be such a confusing time for mothers and daughters. I prayed for a baby girl and organised a humanist naming ceremony that I thought was progressive yet pink-themed. Rowan believes gender is a damaging social construct and has changed her name from the one I gave her – Bella – to be less binary. I posted a black square on social media to mark the Black Lives Matter movement being more important than ever; Rowan said anti-racism has become a trend for white people to feel better about themselves. We are a little bewildered.

The idea for this book came about after Rowan recovered from sepsis, during the pandemic. The chaos of 2020 and shock of a life-threatening illness forced us to talk, to reconnect, to understand. Making sense of each other at a time when nothing made sense anchored us and reminded us of the only things that really matter. Our conversations made the ground beneath us feel more solid. Our curiosity in the other was a safety blanket. For the first time since Rowan was much younger, we talked every day, really talked, discovered how different were our perspectives on life, on matters ranging from our class backgrounds to huge movements gaining traction in the world: Black Lives Matter, trans rights, #MeToo. We discussed the global pandemic and climate crisis and threats to democracy. We spoke of gender, knife crime, and police brutality in America. We debated not only the state of geopolitics, economics, and religion, but also about drag, oat milk, knitting, and TikTok.

As Rowan made a slow recovery in hospital and then at home, our words became more urgent, even more important.

I'd curl up next to her in bed for hours, fill my mind with her thoughts, fill hers with mine. On Deliveroo, urbanism, vampire narratives, misogyny, globalisation, consumerism, home décor, drugs and alcohol, divorce, Uber ratings, introversion, make-up, self-harm, baking, housing, freedom, nuclear war, the Royal Family. We argued, too. About activism, feminism, sex work, independence, meat. And about puppies, North Korea, imperialism, and beauty. Through hearing uncomfortable truths, listening, and self-exploration on both our parts, we forged a new understanding of each other and ourselves. In this age of division, of a widening gap between generations and a deep divide in perspectives, we ultimately found joy and humour in the grey areas between us. I felt pregnant with her once more – as if she was growing inside me, in my head instead of my belly. She saw me clearly, too; perhaps for the first time. In delving into the meaning of our own family, we some-how became more tolerant, hopeful, and optimistic about the future of our world. We really, really listened. *I* really, really listened. As a mother and daughter going through the storms of adolescence and peri-menopause as well as a pandemic, exist-ential threats, and a rapidly changing culture, we somehow reconnected.

This traumatic pause at a pivotal moment both in our personal lives and in history was, it turns out, a precursor to a much bigger storm. After sepsis, after the pandemic, when life was returning to normal, mental illness stabbed our relationship in the heart. Rowan's mental health breakdown came from nowhere and caught us both totally unprepared. Our deep-dive conversations morphed into misunderstandings, arguments, and finally silence. It affected her siblings, dad, stepmum, (now) stepdad, grandparents, teachers, neighbours, and friends, but it took me down entirely. I spent the best part of eighteen months feeling like I could not leave the house in case she hurt herself, and lying awake all night listening for sounds of her pacing up and down, up and down, or of the bathroom door or the kitchen cupboards. I hid the knives, the lighters, the scissors; but of course nursing taught me that if she really wanted to hurt herself, she would find a way. I remember going into her bedroom one day, searching for anything that might be harmful and coming across her sewing kit from her younger years, sitting on her bedroom floor, and looking through the contents for needles to remove. I found a small tapestry she'd made when she was in a textiles phase. I pictured her younger self, my quirky, wonderful daughter, sitting for hours with swatches of different fabric, plotting what she would design and make. I took out anything sharp, and then I wept.

Parenting a mentally unwell teenager is a lonely place. People didn't really understand. Not really. How could they? I would never have believed such pain and worry was possible had I not experienced it. A grief for your child and grief for their future. She lost herself as a daughter for a while, and I lost myself as a mum. But there was community, even in this. I discovered not only that we weren't alone but also that literally dozens of friends were experiencing something similar. A friend's daughter spent a year in an eating disorder treatment unit. Another was repeatedly hospitalised for self-harming. A friend's son, who was always top of his class, found himself unable to leave his bedroom for months on end, and he lost his school place. Nurse friends in A&E echoed what I was experiencing at home. 'We've never seen anything like it', one told me. 'Mental illness is the number one thing that society should be concerned about; until we invest in our young people's mental health, this dire situation is going to get worse. Kids are in so much emotional pain they are dying.'

What was happening to our children? Why, post pandemic, when things were returning to 'normality', were young people falling apart in such catastrophic ways?

We were lucky. After around eighteen months of utter chaos, Rowan's mental health began to even out a fraction, and, therefore, mine did as well. As we clawed our way back, we began talking once more, sometimes in different ways. Humour helped. As did strange, weird quirks. Forgiveness, on both our parts, was everything. It was almost impossible to navigate what was illness, what was simply teenage drama, and what was, frankly, just being a bit of an arsehole – on both sides. But somehow, by communicating in sometimes inventive ways, checking our own behaviour and responses, apologising to each other, and forgiving ourselves for our mistakes, we built a bond strong enough to withstand the darkest of times. Through the tsunami of mental health issues, we discovered much about each other, and ourselves.

It turned out that even the worst of all times can be a gift . . .

This book is about surviving generational storms. It's about what it means to be women, and how no mother and daughter live apart, no matter the distance between them.

A LETTER TO MY DAUGHTER

Dear Bella,

I am giving you this letter on your eighteenth birthday, but that's a long way off. Today, you are just two weeks old. I am writing this with you curled up like a comma on my lap. I can't stop looking at you. I'm obsessed. You yawned! You blinked! You pooped! It's incredible how these small things are the big things, really. It feels like a miracle, simply watching you sleep. You're so tiny, yet already mighty. You're content and completely happy on my lap, or on my breast, or shoulder, but the moment you're away from me, all hell breaks loose. I feel the same, though I don't shout quite as loudly. I don't want to be away from you for a moment. I can't stop staring at your face, your perfect toes, long arms, piano-player fingers. I have never known love like this. The world has surely never known love like this. Everyone says it, that love for your children is unconditional, and overwhelming, and pure. It is true. I have never felt in my life more human, or humble.

What a gift you are.

I don't know what kind of mother I'll make. I'm impatient, distracted, eccentric, often, like your grandad says, 'away with the fairies'. I hope I don't mess things up too much. You deserve the best mum in the world, and I fear I'll just be about good enough. I'm sorry in advance for everything I get wrong. I hope you can forgive me.

Now you are eighteen, I wonder what kind of person you are, your interests and hobbies, ambitions and dreams. Imagining getting to know you as a woman makes my heart sing. But for now, today, I will smell your head and breathe you in, and sit and watch you a few more minutes. I'm in a state of total awe, full of wonder about the nature of things. This mother–daughter love is surely deeper than the seas and wider than the sky. Your tiny newborn face contains all the possibilities of the universe.

On your eighteenth birthday, I wanted to remind myself, and remind you, of this time at the beginning. The meaning of all of it. Perhaps the meaning of life itself.

You are so loved.

Mum X

CHAPTER ONE

Aftershocks

Mental Health

Christie: Have you lost your mind? I mean, seriously, I am not joking. Have you lost your mind?

Rowan: *Blinks. Takes a drag on a cigarette. Looks confused. She is propped up in bed against a lot of pillows, smoking a cigarette and flicking ash into a shell.*

Christie: Do you think this is normal behaviour? I knew I could smell smoke. It woke me up! It's 2 a.m. It's two o' clock in the morning and you're smoking? You're smoking in bed?

Rowan: I won't burn the house down. Don't worry. I'm not *you*.

Christie: Put the cigarette out. Now.

Rowan: Why?

Christie: You are sixteen years old. Sixteen. You are smoking in bed. It is 2 a.m. There are so many reasons. You've lost it now. Totally lost it.

Rowan: You need to chill. Stress is not good for you.

Christie: You have! You have lost your mind.

Rowan: You're the one screaming.

Christie: I *am* screaming. Of course I'm screaming. You're *smoking.*

Rowan: Fine. I'll put the cigarette out if you feel that strongly about it. But only because I want to. You're not in control of me. I am. Anyway, it's you who always burns the house down. Not me.

Christie

When Rowan was around seven years old, and my son was four, I set fire to our kitchen. I'd been half asleep. I was working all the hours as a nurse, doing eighty-hour weeks, and even then had to buy groceries with a credit card. I was finally home, and, after putting the kids to bed, incoherent with exhaustion. I'd turned on the gas, and put the kettle on top of the fire, busying myself with tidying up. We'd earlier had a stove kettle that whistled like a screeching train when hot enough, and I was on autopilot, waiting for the sound. I was dog-tired. My bones ached. It was all I could really do to stay upright. I leant against the wall and briefly closed my eyes. First there was a strange metallic odour, then the smoke alarm, and, very quickly, orange flames. My son, Tay, ran down the stairs, bolted into the kitchen, and found me soaking a tea towel to throw over the sparking, melting plastic kettle.

'Get Mummy's phone', I said, 'and stand by the door.'

He zoomed around, focused on the task. I threw the wet towel over the fire, but it seemed to jump rather than extinguish. I turned the oven off and ran more cold water into a vase. Electric fires . . . I racked my brain for any kind of prior training. I'd been a nurse for some decades and had to attend yearly fire safety lectures, which I now cursed myself for not listening to. The kitchen filled with smoke and an unnatural sweet rotting smell. I wet another towel and shouted for Tay to call 999.

But, somehow, this wet towel worked.

It was over as quickly as it had begun. A fizzing sound, and my heartbeat pounding, streaks of blackened soot shooting up behind the oven. No more flames.

I rushed to my son and cancelled the phone call, opened the windows and door, and set him outside in the cold night; a

No Filters

welcome frost was landing on us, the opposite of fire. We took in giant breaths, almost biting the air.

It was then that I looked across the road and saw my daughter standing on the opposite side. She was holding her two favourite cuddly toys and observing us. She had a big coat on, I noticed, and shoes.

In the mad rush of trying to put out the fire, I'd assumed she was ignoring our shouts. That she was upstairs with a pillow over her head, trying to sleep.

But Rowan had sensed something was very wrong. She'd always had an incredible sixth sense. Perhaps inherited, I often wondered, from my dad's mum, who was a spiritualist and regularly talked to the dead. Rowan had apparently heard me shouting, crept downstairs to find commotion and panic, and smelled burning. She had retrieved her two top toys, put on her duffle coat and shoes, and walked outside, standing as far away as possible, in case, she said later, *you burned the house down*.

She has *always* been a survivor.

I'm relying on that.

'Can you collect Rowan please? It's pastoral care at the school. We're just a bit worried about her . . . She seems manic.'

'Manic? What do you mean?'

'I think it's best you come in?'

The first night I realised that something was seriously wrong with Rowan, with *us,* was long after the pandemic. We'd been through lockdown. She'd *survived* urosepsis, a life-threatening infection. My daughter was as resilient as ever. Both of our mental health felt fragile, like everyone's, but we'd made it, and this was the other side. By now, Rowan had sailed through her GCSE exams with flying colours. Her future was bright. The world was waking up, like Sleeping Beauty after a long, long sleep, and the air fizzed with possibilities. Rowan, like all her friends, bolted into being sixteen with enthusiasm and joy.

Everything changed suddenly. A few nights earlier, I'd found her smoking in bed, propped up on her pillows, without a care in the world. I'd put it down to teenage recklessness, poor impulse control, and an immature frontal lobe. Bad behaviour. Fairly normal. I grounded her and confiscated her cigarettes.

But she'd been off since then. Moodier. Snappy. She was a character much like I am, who would explode suddenly, then calm down afterwards, holding no grudges. But there was no calm. And the day before, I'd gone into her room and found a 6-foot painting she'd done on her wall during the night, of a skeleton. It was an incredible painting, and Rowan was born creative, but it was disturbing, too, a million miles away from the rainbows and unicorns she'd painted as a young child; it was also odd that she'd been up all night, painting on her bedroom walls. Still, I thought, as I drove to the school, she'd be hormonal, perhaps overtired, maybe getting a virus. 'Manic' was an odd word for the office to use to describe a sick child, but I wasn't overly anxious.

I arrived at the school to find her altered. Her eyes were different. Wild. Unhinged. Dark. She looked at me but didn't seem to recognise me at all. She looked possessed.

I quizzed her in the car. What had she taken? Surely, this was drugs. There was no other explanation. Drugs were rife in every direction at her age. My children had told me stories of schoolmates regularly smoking weed before school and taking ketamine in parks, as if this was standard practice for many teens. Rowan denied taking drugs, of course, like any self-respecting teenager, but the more she spoke, the more worried I became. Her words were not right. In the wrong order, somehow. She talked about time and feeling like the wind.

'What do you mean, the wind?'

She laughed, but her face looked tearful as if her insides and outsides no longer matched. Her body was tense and her fists clenched.

'I plan to photosynthesise', she said. 'You wouldn't understand.'

At home, she became even stranger. Even more erratic. She sobbed uncontrollably. I phoned 111, despite knowing already what they would say. I didn't want to admit I knew the truth.

The nurse on the other end of the phone talked to Rowan and I listened outside the door as Ro said no, she wasn't suicidal, but she did want to jump on a train to Brighton, and go to the beach and die there, be absorbed by the sand until nothingness. Then she slumped onto the floor and rocked back and forth, howling. 'I want to die', she said. 'I just want to die.'

At that point, I was praying it was drugs. Let it be drugs, and, most of all, let it be temporary.

We arrived in A&E, Rowan was taken to a stripped-bare room and our journey began. Rowan was clearly unwell, and totally lost. She was desperate for a diagnosis, a language for what was happening. I was extremely reluctant for that to happen. In my career, I'd seen too many people suffer stigma, discrimination, and hopelessness, and I was entirely convinced our Western medicalised model of psychiatry did as much harm as good. But everything was suddenly dangerous. She was in agony, that was clear. Her thoughts raced and then fell into darkness. Mine did, too. What if she hurts herself, intentionally or not, my baby girl? What if she doesn't come back to me? Ends up on medications that dampen and dull her? She had blood tests (negative to drugs but that didn't mean she hadn't taken some) and talked to many, many doctors. They were kind but asked the wrong questions: *Have you been sleeping? Eating? How is school? Can you concentrate? How're things at home? Any worries?*

Eventually, a doctor listened. Properly listened. She told him how sad she felt. How hopeless. That her eyesight was now perfect. Twenty-twenty vision. And she no longer needed the glasses she'd always worn.

The rest of the night, she paced. Up and down and up and down, head flicking thoughts from side to side, occasionally putting her hands to her ears to stop the relentless noise.

I followed the doctor out of the room, desperate. 'She seems psychotic. What's wrong with her?' I thought of my school friend who had died by suicide aged twenty-one after experiencing delusions and strange thoughts out of the blue, and displaying erratic behaviour. How desperate he must have felt. Words echoed in my head – phrases, conditions, serious illnesses that the wider mental health conversation seemingly ignored:

Schizo-affective Disorder
Bipolar
Borderline Personality Disorder

I prayed again to all the gods I could think of that Rowan's condition was drug-related. But then I imagined my child addicted to heroin. Nursing is a terrible gift. I know however bad, there can always be worse. Always.

'Let's take a breath', the doctor said. 'It could be any number of things; so we'll keep her safe here and monitor her after she's rested. If it is psychosis, and again it's a major 'if', it's important we have this early information, and even then, it can have several causes . . .'

We were sent home a day later with a waiting list appointment at Child and Adolescent Mental Health Services (CAMHS), which did not reassure me at all. The Royal College of Paediatrics and Child Health (RCPCH) reported that in May 2023 the waiting list for CAMHS was the highest it had ever been and had increased 39 per cent in just two years. Rowan was now one of the 403,995 children who were waiting to be seen for mental health support, and the RCPCH discovered 17,991 children were waiting for more than a year to be seen.

So many families in crisis, like us, armed with nothing but a leaflet that advised to lock away anything sharp, including knives and scissors, and hide all medications, and provided a list of emergency numbers to call if Rowan was suicidal or tried to harm herself. She was prescribed a sedative as a temporary measure, a sort of chemical restraint. Finally, she slept.

I called her dad, but I didn't know what to say other than that she was mentally unwell and I didn't know what was wrong with her. Then I went into her bedroom and sat on her bed, watching her breathe. Her face even in sleep was etched with pain.

'*Come back to me*', I whispered. '*Please come back to me.*'

Rowan

I sat on the floor next to Rosemary's dog, Pebble, and told her everything. Like all my friends, I spent a lot of time here in the pastoral care office, probably more than in my actual lessons. The office was a calm place. A sanctuary. There were bean bags, cushions, and blankets, a kettle and cups for coffee or hot chocolate, a glass jar full of marshmallows. On the walls were postcards and motivational quotes and photographs of animals – the teacher's pets mostly and a random turtle – all pinned to colourful mood boards. There were gay and trans pride flags everywhere.

Rosemary knew every single detail of our lives. God knows why she let us go in there and have her therapise us – she didn't get paid anywhere near enough to be dealing with that. But she always welcomed us anyway, with our steady stream of the terror and sadness of being sixteen. She listened to all our worries and antics, and, unlike my mum, she never ever judged. Sometimes she'd give us advice, but mostly she just gave us hot chocolate, and she had this wide-open smile that made the worst of things seem less awful.

That day, I was a bit hysterical. My hormonal mood swings had, somehow, become delusions, but I didn't know that. I could hear my voice clearly. I felt like I was the truest I'd ever been and amplified. I couldn't stop talking. Rambling. Usually, I'd chat with Rosemary, have a cry and a hot chocolate, then feel a fraction better, and go back to lessons.

'I think that time has no meaning', I said, 'and sometimes I feel like the wind, not really human. You know?'

She stopped stirring the hot chocolate and frowned at me. 'Rowan, you seem a bit manic. Have you taken anything?'

I shook my head, but even my head-shaking felt a bit weird. Quicker somehow. I was hyper-aware that my body was just a shell I was living in and had no real connection to me. Like my head didn't belong to my body or I wasn't really there. I thought about my friends and asked Rosemary where they were and if any of them were off school. They were always off school with mental health issues, and I hadn't seen them. I was one of the calmer ones in my friendship group, because everyone my age is a bit crazy post pandemic. Plus, this was art school. We were the generation who all wanted to die but still had a twenty-step skincare routine. Around once a month, my best friend, Chloe was taken from school to A&E by ambulance, India went every couple of months, Kate never had to and Jaz lived in the hospital, as did Rose.

That day, it was my turn.

The process for getting help for mental illness is strange. You are suddenly surrounded by adults offering no diagnosis but instead a step-by-step plan. It was suggested to me by various people over the coming days that the following solutions might cure my out-of-control brain:

Taking a warm bath
Listening to my favourite music
Putting my hands into a bowl of ice
Watching my favourite film
Some gentle exercise
Making a nice cup of tea
A sensory box – filled with different smells and textures
My favourite chocolate

Meanwhile, my mum had been told to hide the kitchen knives and lock away the paracetamol.

I was told that my sadness and my madness were most likely caused by smoking weed, as weed can trigger something that causes psychosis; but that didn't feel right. Doctors then suggested I had anxiety, which didn't make sense either as I didn't ever get stressed out or worry – I don't see the point. Also, anxiety, to my knowledge, did not explain that I thought I was the wind. Literally, the wind. The next pseudo-diagnosis, 'low mood disorder', came from a psychiatrist in A&E and it annoyed me, not because it was untrue – my mood was low, and I had experienced suicidal thoughts plenty of times – but the wording was a bit insulting to me. It sounded like I'd bought Tesco's own brand of depression.

In the end, nobody could label me or tell me what was wrong. It was nameless, existing only in dingy shadows. I had appointment after appointment that my mum would drive me to and from, trying so hard to not ask me questions or antagonise me in any way, which, of course, she did all the time. The final assessment I had before starting psychotherapy and coming off the medication that made me sleep about eighteen hours a day was with a psychiatrist named George, who looked about my age and seemed to me like the kind of guy who played rugby and drank pints of his own piss for a laugh. I had stopped going to school by then. Most days, I just cried in bed, or slept, or scrolled through TikTok looking at other girls who were also mentally unwell. A lot of people posted from psychiatric hospitals, their faces bloody with cuts, foreheads covered with large plasters.

We went to the CAMHS centre fairly often, a soulless building. Mum said we were so lucky getting seen quickly, but it didn't feel that way. The waiting area was full of dead-eyed teenage girls and hyper-cheerful mothers, sitting next to each other but a million miles apart. The room we sat in had a large table with a box of tissues on it, which my mum and I ignored. I had been in a faraway place. My mum didn't know where I was, and nor did the psychiatrist. I once heard Mum say that psychiatry is a like a blind man in a dark room looking for a black cat that doesn't really exist.

George looked at me, searching for the cat that doesn't exist, but I ignored him and instead screamed at my mum. She'd said something that pissed me off, and we both built. Her face was puffed up from crying.

'I told you I didn't want to be here!' I screamed. 'This is your fault. I get it from you.'

She should have been calm. Taken deep breaths. She was the grown-up. But she screamed back at me. We were both so broken neither had any sense of politeness anymore. We hadn't slept in a long time.

Mental illness, it turns out, is completely contagious.

We screamed and shouted at each other as though we were the only ones in the room, or in this world. 'I've had enough Ro. Enough. I understand you're not well, but you are also A DICK.'

She's a writer, so you'd think she could use better words. But it could have been worse, I guess. 'I am a giant dick because I take after you! You should never have been a mother! Ever, ever!'

We were sword fighting with words until one of us was fatally wounded. Today, I landed the final blow. Still, she continued to scream and shout and I shouted back, and neither of us noticed the psychiatrist back slowly out of the room until he was at the door.

We turned our heads at the same time and stared at him.

'I think I see the issue now', George whispered. Then he left.

My mum and I looked at the door a while, then at each other. And somehow, despite everything, maybe *because* of everything, we both began to laugh.

★

My mum feels in the extremes, too. I get that from her and it's mostly a gift, but that combined with my father's inability to process emotion fucked me over. Learning that was strange and painful, an undoing of myself. My mum had her own peri-menopausal madness to deal with at the same time, and for an entire dark year, we both got tangled up in each other's minds and moods. So much of what we carry and how we process belongs not to us but to our parents, and their parents, and theirs. But whatever was going on with my mental health, I feel calmer now and better, much more in control of my life, and my future. I understand that I don't need to inherit everyone's issues. I get to choose my own.

Now I'm eighteen and on the other side of this, and with hindsight and recovery, I'm reflecting on the last few years. Like for so many other young women, it was not during but after the pandemic that things fell apart. Being a sixteen-year-old girl is always the worst, but there is something particular to this time that made it dangerous. Mum says we don't have any answers as to what caused my breakdown, but I think living is enough of a reason for a mental collapse. Maybe I was mentally ill. Maybe I'm very sensitive. Maybe I'm really angry. And maybe, just maybe – given the state of the world – that is entirely appropriate. I was not the only person suffering from mental illness after the pandemic. There were millions of teenagers just like me out there feeling like I was – totally lost. I hope this book helps them know that they are not alone. There's a way back.

CONVERSATIONS

GET ME A HAMMER

Tay: *Whispering.* Rowan asked me for a hammer.

Christie: Hi, darling. Do you want to watch this with me? It's a documentary but it's honestly so interesting. About this orca at SeaWorld . . . Think you'd like it.

Tay: *Whispering.* Mum, did you hear me? Ro asked me for a hammer.

Christie: What are you talking about? *Pauses documentary.*

Tay: Rowan. She's upstairs in her bedroom and she asked me to come in and then asked me for a hammer. She was laughing, so I don't think she wants to hit anyone with it.

Christie: Why does she want a hammer?

Tay: I'm not sure. But in light of everything recent, I thought I should mention it.

Christie: Yes, I'm glad you did! OK I'll go up. Wait, you didn't give a hammer to her?

Tay: Yes. I gave her a hammer.

Christie: --

Tay: Sorry, Mum. I should have probably checked first.

Christie: That's OK. *Running towards stairs.*

CHAPTER TWO

Nature–Nurture

Inheritance

Maternal Grandma: She's unusual like you were.

Christie: What do you mean?

Maternal Grandma: Well, you spent a decade under the table, a sheet covering it, and did a new project every week. Bird-watching, astronomy, anatomy. You had a new notebook every week and a load of library books. You made Tom do the projects with you. Bless him, he just wanted to go out on his bike.

Christie: I sat under a sheet learning about astronomy instead of playing? Poor Tom.

Maternal Grandma: Yes. Then there were the car number plates.

Christie: What number plates?

Maternal Grandma: You memorised number plates. In the local area. You would stop on the way to nursery and suddenly say, MCT6 8NY is missing, or something. Really weird.

Christie: I remembered the number plates of cars? How old was I?

Maternal Grandma: I can't remember. Really little. Anyway, you grew out of all that stuff.

Christie: Or masked it. Did you get me assessed?

Maternal Grandma: Assessed for what? Lots of kids do things like that. Apart from the obsessive projects, maybe. You were clever, that's all. You were totally fine.

Christie

When Rowan began experiencing mental health issues, I searched for clues and began questioning both genetics and inheritance. Had I passed on something I wasn't even aware that I had myself? I agonised over nurture – as well as nature. Was my parenting good enough? Did I make too many mistakes? I kept thinking of the poem 'This Be the Verse' by Philip Larkin; it played over and over in my head during Rowan's adolescence, the line about our parents all fucking us up in their own individual ways, giving us their own issues and extras, too.

I gave Rowan some extras, for sure, and not only by nature but by nurture, too. I went back to work as a nurse when she was five months old, much to the horror of my own parents who expected me to stay at home, at least until she was school-age. 'Why can't her dad stay at home with her?' I'd often say, only to be met with confusion – a baffled expression on my mum's face that was often followed by conversations about how the first five years at home with me and my brother were the best time of her life. My mum couldn't understand why I would leave a baby with strangers in order to work.

'With childcare costs, it makes no financial sense', my mum reminded me. A fact which itself says everything about motherhood and the value – or not – of women in our patriarchal system. But she bit her tongue on many occasions, too. As a child protection social worker, and, therefore, expert on attachment theory, she understood much more than I did about potential, even unintentional, developmental harm.

You can't have it all, it turns out. Or rather, women can't.

Perhaps Ro's breakdown was because I'd given her attachment issues by leaving her so very young in childcare and working long hours? Although I did not know as much as my mum, I'd studied child development, and particularly attachment theory, for many years at nursing school. I understood John Bowlby, the renowned psychiatrist and psychoanalyst who developed attachment theory regarding the importance of a secure and consistent attachment to the primary caregiver in early childhood and even babyhood. Bowlby theorised that inconsistencies or disruptions in early attachments could lead to mental health problems. But still, when Rowan was only two years old, I began an MA in Creative Writing at the University of East Anglia and travelled back and forth between London and Norwich. I was permanently distracted. The reading list was eye-watering. I would put Rowan in the bath and watch her make Father Christmas beards with the bubbles as I read sitting on the toilet seat. There was no way of getting through all of the books in the reading list. I worked out that you can pretty much understand a book, and a writer, from the first three and the last chapters. I didn't consider that mirrored human life: the fact that I was mid book, fully formed, but Rowan was in her crucial first three chapters. In addition to doing the MA, and writing my first novel, I worked part-time, nursing children who had life-limiting illnesses. I was too often preoccupied. Always exhausted.

Rowan, inevitably, didn't start talking until she was almost four. We had a secret language. I didn't even realise that we were talking gobbledegook, let alone that I was most likely contributing to the delay in her language development, until a friend pointed it out.

'I can understand her perfectly well', I said.

Rowan stood in front of me, dressed, as she always was until she began to question the structural basis of gender, in her yellow sateen Belle ball gown from *Beauty and the Beast*, a tiara, and dress-up plastic heeled shoes that clicked as she walked around the house and twirled in front of the mirror.

'What is it?' I asked her. 'What do you need?'

Then I heard it: 'Geem any tapar ggguuubenfhsgfucusb sigfbdngcd.'

My friend raised her eyebrows. Her son was only five and already learning French.

'She's asking for an orange and if I can peel it.'

My friend laughed, but then stood astonished as I got an orange from the fruit bowl, cut it into segments and handed it to Ro on a melamine plate. She waited patiently then took the plate and sat down, demonstrating that this was exactly what she was expecting.

I've often wondered about this time. Could I really understand her language? Did I know instinctively what she wanted? Or did I simply seem confident enough to her that she trusted whatever I gave her was exactly what she'd been looking for? Whatever the driving factor, she felt seen and heard by me, and that was all that mattered.

Being seen and being heard, however, was often very hard for Ro when, as an artist, I was hyper-focused on work. I was selfish to imagine my being a writer wouldn't impact my kids. Even when I was physically present, I was too often in my head, in my made-up imaginary worlds. Writing, like nursing, is the fabric of me. I couldn't imagine a life where I was not writing. I do not want to. But living a creative life and balancing that with the humdrum of parenting small children . . . something always had to give. Being a writer involves much sacrifice, and as a single parent, I was making sacrifices on their behalf as well as my own.

But whatever the struggles of having a writer mum, there were good parts to it, too. Rowan inherited my creativity. She became more and more imaginative year on year. I had a phone call from her primary school wishing us the best of luck with our new life in LA. We were not, to my knowledge, moving to LA anytime soon. When she was around nine, I took Rowan to the seaside, where she encountered a mermaid who later became her friend, as real to her as any other friend. There was also a stranger side to this imagination; Ro never seemed able to separate fact from fiction. She'd remember things that didn't happen with such clarity that it was impossible to convince her the memory was not right. By the time she began secondary school, it was clear she was wired unusually, and more than likely, like I am. When this quirky way of seeing the world collided with teenage development, her creativity took her to dark places.

'I wanted to give you a call about your daughter. She's fine, don't worry, just a few concerns.' Another day, another teacher. This time English. Rowan was thirteen. 'She has been writing some really dark things. We're quite worried about her mental health.'

'I'm not following. You're her English teacher? Has she handed in something concerning?'

'Not handed in, no. During lessons. She's been writing poetry during English lessons and not following what we're doing.'

'What's she writing? Sorry, poetry?'

'Yes, poetry. Incredibly dark. Actually, pretty good poetry, but she's not focusing on class and instead she's writing poetry. Dark poetry about death and suicide and love. A poem about bones and flesh. That kind of thing.'

'I'm sorry, I'm still not quite following. You're saying that she's writing good poetry, though dark, in English class, and this is a problem?'

'Well, yes. She's not following the curriculum. We're worried about her mental health. Perhaps she needs to see someone.'

'Did you ask her about the poems?'

'Yes. She said she likes writing poetry. She's been told to put her poetry away in class and concentrate on the lessons. But other teachers have found she's doing the same.'

'She's writing poetry in school, in class? For fun?'

'Yes. I know you must feel worried. It's very disturbing poetry.'

'Isn't all poetry disturbing? I mean isn't that the point of poetry? To disturb?'

At our first CAMHS appointment, Ro did not speak at all. Every ten minutes or so she'd shrug, slowly, as if moving her shoulders was painful. She was an empty shell of a human being.

Eventually, she opted to wait outside and nodded a fraction that it was OK for me to talk with the team. I was holding back tears. I hadn't slept in weeks, instead lying awake and worrying about her all night, listening out for every single tiny noise. We still didn't know what was wrong. Or how to fix it.

'Has it ever been suggested that Rowan might be neurodiverse, have ADHD, for example?' Her therapist, a young, slightly terrified-looking woman, asked while scribbling in a large notebook.

I shook my head. Neither of us had ever been diagnosed as neurodivergent. But then I thought back. When she was in primary school, I was told Rowan was cartwheeling instead of concentrating. She had piano lessons for a year before I discovered she played with her feet instead of her hands. She explained things through dance instead of words. I imagined she was a bit different. Like I am. A bit of a square peg in a round hole world. A creative, like me. Was I wrong?

The King's Fund found that in 2017, rates of probable mental disorders affected 10.1 per cent of young people aged seventeen to nineteen years. That figure in 2023 was 23.3 per cent. Nobody can explain exactly why there is this massive, alarming increase in mental illness in adolescents, though the pandemic and social media are often cited as factors. Neurodiversity, or, at least, diagnoses of neurodivergence in both children and adults, seems to be growing at an even faster rate. The term 'neurodiverse' was coined by an Australian academic, Judy Singer, in 1998, to describe the idea of neurological diversity and develop ideas for a social movement of neurological minorities. She described that it was when she became a parent in 1987 that she began thinking deeply about the complexities of human psychology and traits people inherit from their parents. Singer describes that 'after her daughter was diagnosed with Asperger's at the age of nine, Singer began to recognise certain traits in herself'.[1]

During my nursing career, I looked after hundreds of children with severe learning disabilities; many of the children had neurological disabilities so acute that it affected their everyday lives in every possible way. They did not reach developmental milestones. They needed speech and language therapy, and special education. Some were non-verbal or had challenging behaviours, others were incontinent or unable to feed themselves. Neurodiversity, I'd always thought, doesn't need pathologising. I felt wired a little unusually but had never seen any need to seek a diagnosis. I was in a privileged place of functioning in everyday life and having some understanding of my habits and behaviours. Birkbeck University of London's Centre for Neurodiversity at Work describes the unique skills and talents that people with neurodiverse conditions bring to the workforce, including ability to hyper-focus, creativity, innovative thinking, and strength in processing details.[2] Being a bit neuro-spicy, whether self-diagnosed, diagnosed, or not, felt to me a lot like a superpower. But I learnt that it certainly doesn't feel like that to everyone.

Ro's therapist told me that many girls came in experiencing mental health problems with co-occurring neurodevelopmental conditions, or misdiagnosis, and that once named, conditions like ADHD can be easy to treat with medication. 'Many, many people with neurodiverse conditions need support, as often it affects every aspect of their lives.'

Should I have had Rowan assessed for ADD, ADHD, autism or other neurodiversity at a young age? Should I have had my own assessments? I have a handful of friends who were dealing with teenage daughters struggling with behaviour and emotions only to discover that their children are autistic, or have ADHD, or both; and then the mothers get diagnosed, too – a great surprise to Generation X, who have always seemingly laboured under the rhetoric of 'just get on with it'. WE ARE FINE. Women have been masking, and often suffering, for years. The *Guardian* reports that 15 to 20 per cent of the population is thought to be neurodivergent.[3] But girls – and women – have been woefully underdiagnosed. *The Journal of Attention Disorders* presented an article named *Miss Diagnosis – A Systemic Review of ADHD in Adult Women* that highlighted just how many women seeking treatment for mood and emotional problems may have ADHD, which can cause low self-esteem, feelings of failure, guilt, and inadequacy.[4] The National Autistic Society reports that the most recent data show that boys and men are three times more likely to be diagnosed with autism compared to girls and women.[5] Women and girls are far more likely to mask and camouflage symptoms.

Alongside this reported underdiagnosis, at least in a clinical sense, there is real fear among some parents who worry that self-diagnosis of neurodiversity is becoming popular among some young teens. A psychiatrist friend is worried we risk going from stigmatising to glamorising, and what pressure might that cause, both to overstretched services and for people who need serious help. But the more I discover and read about neurodiversity and think about myself, and Ro, the greater number of lightbulbs go off in my head.

Mental health is a soup of nature, nurture, environment, personality, and even luck. There is no doubt that neurodevelopmental biology and childhood attachment patterns, both nature *and* nurture, are key ingredients, and there are many more, too.

'Do you want to try and get a diagnosis?' I asked Ro. She was sitting on the floor leaning against the washing machine. She no longer sat in chairs. I had no idea why, but I picked my battles, and this one was not important. 'I mean, to see if you have ADHD. Because if so, medication might be helpful.'

'Not really.'

'This is not about mental health but neurodiversity and medication can be useful. The more I read up about it the more I suspect I've gifted you something.'

'It's not that I'm not that bothered', she said. 'But all my friends are waiting for diagnoses, and they've been waiting years; so it seems a bit of a waste of time to me. You should get checked out though. I mean if you want.'

'Maybe one day. It's not a priority for me at that moment.' I didn't tell her that my only priority at that moment was Rowan, but that was true. I didn't feel able to leave the house in case she harmed herself in some way. It was all-consuming.

Rowan began to cry. She often did, and from nowhere. I sat next to her. But she moved away.

'Talk to me', I said. 'What is making you upset? The possible ADHD thing?'

She changed then, from sad to angry. The flip of a switch. 'I don't fucking care about neurodiversity. That's not the reason for this. I'm mentally ill, and I've been mentally ill for literally years, and you didn't see it.'

She held her head in her hands and started to rock and sob as if her brain was on fire. She was right. I did not see it. I could never have imagined my daughter being in such psycho-logical pain.

Eventually, she stopped and took her hands away. I sat still on the floor beside her. When she was a baby, or a toddler, and screaming, I used to try and slow down my breathing, in the hope that eventually she would match my calm. That is not so easy with a teenager, but it is just as important. She was a lost little girl, hidden in an almost adult body.

I didn't talk. I simply sat, and breathed, and waited for Ro's shoulders to rise and fall in time with my own.

Rowan

Mum says that having a mentally unwell teenager is holding a mirror up to your own parenting and your own genetics. 'It turns out', she told me, 'that if you are parenting a mentally ill, emotionally unstable teenager, chances are you are mentally ill and emotionally unstable in some way, too. The apple never falls far from the tree. I worry that I've passed on some unusual wiring. At least you didn't inherit my short legs.' She coughed and apologised.

'It's not that deep', I told her. But I could tell she didn't believe me. I read this story once about telepathy and I remember thinking that it was a learnt skill. After all, I could read Mum's mind at all times. But when I became a teenager, I understood this only happened in one direction. I always knew what Mum was thinking, but she could never guess what was happening in my thoughts. *The apple never falls far from the tree*, I was thinking in agreement with her, *but the tree can't help what kind of tree it is*. An apple tree can't decide to be a weeping willow. It's an apple tree.

At my first CAMHS appointment, they asked me lots of questions. Some of them were clearly about looking for clues for what else, apart from mental health stuff, might be going on with me. They asked me if I fidgeted a lot, found it hard to sit still or concentrate, and talked a lot about black and white thinking. They asked if I'd ever had an autism and ADHD assessment. I hadn't, and I didn't want to go after one. Not that I didn't want to know about my brain, but I had friends who waited four years to get assessed for neurodiversity, and that seemed like a lot of effort. Maybe I'll try to get assessed at some point, but then it didn't bother me if I was neuro-spicy or not. I realise this a privilege in itself. Lots of my friends needed treatment and support so badly and were not getting the help they deserved for neurodiverse conditions. But I liked the way my brain worked, most of the time; and also, I could clearly see that some parts of me were just like Mum.

I remember Mum coming home from a paediatric ward and telling me this story. She said a kid came in after a minor car accident; he seemed drowsy, unable to focus. He had a laugh, she said, like a machine gun. The staff worried if the drowsiness and strange laugh might indicate a brain injury, and they ordered tons of tests and scans – but then his dad arrived on the ward. 'This man walked in', Mum laughed, 'a bit dazed-looking and his voice sounded a bit like a machine gun going off.' She smiled and told me how happy the little boy was to see his dad. They were like mirrors of each other. 'We cancelled the CT scan', she said.

Aside from enquiring about a slightly off-key way of looking at the world, working out if I was a bit neuro-spicy, the CAMHS team asked a lot of questions about my early years, especially about my relationship with Mum. It was like being interviewed by a team of detectives. I had a pretty happy early childhood overall, but like all childhoods, there were also challenges.

Mum was a single parent from when my brother and I were four and seven years old, and with that, at times, I inevitably had unreasonable responsibilities. I remember her working all the time, and even when not working, she was writing, living in her own head. Sometimes, she would have to leave at 5 a.m. and wouldn't be back till around 11 p.m. Each morning, I would sneak to the top of the stairs to say bye and watch as she tripped over her shoes or sat on our couch for a few minutes, completely still. She looked as if she was about to run a marathon. I remember cooking for my brother sometimes from around the age of ten and taking two-hour bus journeys to avoid having to ask for train money. Like many older children in single-parent families, I felt short-changed. She wasn't there as much as I wanted.

That I never directed my anger towards my dad, who was

absent for almost my entire childhood, is an uncomfortable truth. At one time, I believed that even his absence, surely, was somehow my mum's fault. Everything was. It was her job to keep me safe.

Suddenly, when I became a teenager, I did not feel at all safe. I didn't know what I was doing, and she sure as shit didn't either. We were both making things up as we went. Realizing that is a terrifying part of growing up..

I played with my brother constantly but don't remember having any friends when I was very young, something I wasn't aware of and wasn't that bothered by. My childhood recollections are blurry, like a story that I was never in; I'm unsure if my memories are true or imagined. I got this from Mum. She lived between the real world and whatever fictional world she was writing about. It's not that nothing was real, more that *everything* was real.

'Blessing', she shouted upstairs one day, 'dinner's ready.'

I ignored her and looked in the mirror. It sounds strange but I think I was checking that I had somehow not turned into Blessing. Blessing was a character in the novel Mum had written. She was around my age, twelve at the time. Mum said she borrowed language from me sometimes, but in the case of Blessing, who she had invented a decade earlier, she borrowed language from my big sister, Alex. She said twelve-year-old girls had a snappy energy to their words.

'Blessing!'

I came out of the bathroom and shouted over the banister. 'I'm not Blessing. I'm Bella. I'm your REAL daughter.'

It's the first time I remember feeling really angry with Mum.

I clearly remember feeling sad, too, watching Mum sitting on our scratchy grey couch at dawn, staring a moment into the air or with her head in her hands. It was like I felt her feelings, as well as my own, even if she tried to hide them. I remember waiting for her to get home and looking out of my window at the moon, wondering if she was OK. Missing her.

My whole early childhood I considered Mum a friend and admired her. I wanted her magical colour-changing eyes. I wanted to be funny and kind the same way she is. But at some point, I didn't want to be a mirror of Mum anymore. My mum was suddenly not how I imagined a mum should be and nor was our relationship. I felt something was wrong with me, and my favourite place became my room and my least favourite person, my mum. I didn't want to be different, like she was. I wanted to be 'normal' and her to be the same as other mums. I wished she was more 'motherly'. I wished she had spent more time with me and been more present, even if she did have to work all the hours. I wish, I wish, I wish.

I remember having this friend whose mum was there after school every day. She dropped whatever she was doing and sat down with us both, asking questions about the day and our friends, and listened as she drank a cup of tea, not in a rush, spending a long time. Then my friend's dad would turn up at teatime and he'd sit down with us, too, and ask my friend about her day, and they'd eat toad in the hole together and talk, then have pudding on a Monday – unheard of in my house.

Meanwhile, my mum would be shouting at the news, or suggesting we go to a second-hand bookshop and smell the books, or reading poetry to my brother and me, scrambling around for a makeshift dinner as she'd forgotten to go grocery shopping. She played jazz trumpet loud enough that our neighbours banged on the wall and did random activities like aerial trapeze or build a 'pub shed'. On election nights, she'd bring a quilt into the living room and literally camp, and try to get us to stay up all night, bribing us with popcorn to watch American politics instead of Harry Potter. We'd claim tiredness and point out that we had school the next day. 'Some things are more important than school', she'd say.

Even holidays were unusual. While my friend and her parents went all-inclusive to Tenerife and enjoyed a week relaxing by the pool, we were in Croatia during a forest fire, and Mum borrowed a boat and sped out towards the flames. We spent a day under the airplane that was water-bombing, scooping sea water so dangerously close to us the boat almost capsized, as she talked about aerial firefighting, the climate emergency, and the magic of the sea. Or Egypt, when she took me to some remote village and somehow convinced a local fisherman to take us out to the deep blue sea, where the fisherman pissed over the side of the boat, and Mum insisted we dive into the freezing water to swim with dolphins. I was young. I remember crying. It was too much. She was too much.

At least it was never boring. But sometimes, I just wanted her to be there after school, making me a jam sandwich or actually getting excited about Sports Day.

Having a writer as a mum was an odd experience. Maybe she is neuro-spicy, and maybe I am, but sometimes, I wonder if all writers think like she does. Novelists at least. Every year Mum would go into her 'writing pit': just lock herself in her room for about three months like a hibernating bear. The only time she'd come out would be for coffee. Her diet consisted of anything she could grab while she waited for the kettle to boil; usually pistachios, occasionally yoghurt. She didn't sleep. She'd wake up randomly after an hour or two of sleep with some new genius idea she had to get down, at 3 a.m. I would watch her from the top of the stairs, pacing up and down, coffee in hand, before sitting at the computer and typing ferociously.

After the first draft came the editing. Friends would reappear in our lives, and the schedule was less brutal. Mum was less far-away, and lighter. We loved her friends. Mum collected misfits: other creatives, writers, actors, artists. They exposed me to art, music, culture and, always, politics, but often this bohemian chaos felt like living in a nuthouse. They were each as crazy as they were kind. I had a lot of mentally ill role models, that's for sure.

Growing up in a single-parent, multi-heritage, multi-faith, neuro-spicy household with a creative and unusual mum has shaped me. It took a long time to make sense of it all, but now I think being like Mum is a very good thing. I'm glad she's a bit weird. It made me feel confident that I can be completely my own person. Mum encouraged healthy debate. She gifted me a lifelong love of books and political anger. Mostly, she let me be myself. She was always a terrible dancer and doesn't really understand dance the way I do, but she was there, cheering me on. It's funny because although my memories are of her working really hard and being absent, I also know she spent years driving me around dance classes and schools, sitting in the car in the rain while working on deadlines. When I would come out, she got out of the car every time and demonstrated her infamous 'crab dance', a performance she pulled out at every party, the worst dance moves I've ever seen.

I can now see my earlier views on family structure were a bit warped. I craved normal, but what family is normal, anyway? My friend who had the 'perfect' family, the present and attentive parents, ended up with mental health issues so severe she was repeatedly sectioned and is now estranged from her parents.

My mum wasn't perfect, but she created a home where it was always OK to be different, however that looked. When I told her, around thirteen, that I was Triple bi, she looked confused.

'What do you mean? Triple bi?' Mum was wearing two dressing gowns, I noticed, and leopard print slippers. She spent an extraordinary amount of time in dressing gowns.

'Triple bi', I said. I wanted to shock her. To get a reaction. At thirteen, that drove me. 'Biracial, bisexual, and bipolar.'

Mum's mouth dropped open a fraction, but then she closed it and pressed her lips together. Was she trying not to laugh? She was silent a few seconds, then she smiled and kissed me on the head. 'You do you', she said.

CONVERSATIONS

COSHED

Maternal Grandad: *Opens the front door.* What is that racket? It's one o'clock in the bloody morning. The baby's just gone down. My newborn granddaughter. Stop shouting in the street and go home to your families.

Young Man: It's my mate. There's been a fight. He's been coshed. Everyone's fighting outside the pub.

Christie: What's happening? What do you mean coshed? Should I get an ambulance, Dad?

Young Man: He's hurt badly. Bleeding.

Christie: I'll phone an ambulance.

Maternal Grandad: Don't. I'll check it out. You go and make sure Bella is OK.

Christie: She's fine. Fast asleep.

A group of angry young men are walking down the road towards the man outside our house.

Maternal Grandad: *Closes door, leans against it. Whispers.* Get me a fucking hammer.

Christie: Absolutely not.

CHAPTER THREE

Almond Mum

Disordered Eating

Rowan: What *is* that? In the toilet? Looks like a nappy . . . Wait, what are you eating?

Christie: I'm testing my gut microbiome.

Rowan: Gut what? That looks like playdough. Ew. Gross. Why?

Christie: It's not the best. *Retches.*

Rowan: *Retches.*

Christie: It's a special cookie. I eat two, then record my gut transit time. Hence, the nappy thing in the toilet.

Rowan: You're what?

Christie: *Holds up a testing kit.* It's a great new study where they have done a ton of research showing how we've got diets all wrong. It's not about less food, but more, in order for you to be healthy. For your gut microbes to be diverse. This (*holds up a sterile container*) is for poo, which they then test for a gazillion bacteria. Good and bad ones. Apparently, there's one parasite they test for that some people have, which means they naturally stay slim. Who knew?

Rowan: You want a *parasite* living in you? To stay slim? Let me get this right. You're eating playdough to then shit in a nappy and collect it to send to a lab so they can test you for bacteria?

Christie: Yup. And this contraption is a small needle that sits in my arm for two weeks so I can record my blood sugar after every meal. And no, I don't want a parasite, but it's interesting.

Rowan: You do! You actually want a parasite, I can tell. Your generation have some serious food issues, along with toxic body image. You're shitting in a nappy, eating playdough, and sticking a needle in your arm. Why? Why?

Christie: It's science.

Rowan: It's fucked up, that's what it is.

Christie: Stop swearing. Please. Honestly, it's not about dieting, or body image. The research is there. Gut microbiome diversity is the future.

Rowan: It's cray-cray! But at least one kind of diversity is gaining traction among middle-aged white folk, I guess. *Cracks up.*

Rowan

Thirteen was the peak. We were at the most pliable age and had yet to give much thought to the patriarchy, consumerism, Western body ideals or globalisation. After school each day, I'd go with my three friends to Sophie's house as she lived the closest and her parents cared the least about our being there. We'd spent the last few months doing stupid shit like mixing random ingredients together and eating it for dares, a tablespoon of mustard, vinegar, pepper and mayo, a sprinkle of chilli sauce, and once, a dog biscuit. We laughed hysterically, rolling around on the ground, retching after the magic concoctions, and then watched TV under Sophie's snuggly duvet, drinking Fanta and 7Up, seeing who could burp the loudest. Me, it turns out. I remember the day it changed into something else. A shadow of something passed over us, but I couldn't name what it was. It started with the fitness.

'We're doing a ten-minute abs workout every single day', Sophie announced at school, and Kaley and I both nodded, mesmerised by the idea. It sounded so grown-up. Plus, we wanted a six pack. We ran to her house, to 'burn some extra calories', and lay down like sardines in Sophie's hallway, watching the app she had set up on her new iPhone. It was a nice kind of sore, but it didn't end there. Sophie had a wild-eyed look on her face as she reeled off what were 'good' foods (vegetables, eggs, salad), 'bad' foods (cake, chocolate, ice cream). 'We should try and eat mostly legume', she said. Kaley and I had no idea what legume was, but we nodded anyway. Sounded exotic.

Sophie quickly got obsessed with food. We all agreed that instead of eating only 'good' foods and not the 'bad' foods we loved, we would simply eat a tiny amount, like mice. We'd buy a chocolate bar and divide it into six, eating one portion at lunchtime and one after school, before our abs workout. Then, instead of sitting under Sophie's cuddly duvet and watching films, we would scroll.

We went from fun to anxious almost overnight.

We stopped going to bossmans for snacks every day, Sophie stopped eating bread or anything that resembled carbs, and Kaley, who did not have coeliac disease or even intolerance, acted as if gluten was suddenly the devil.

We scrolled through TikTok and Insta on Sophie's phone until our thumbs hurt as much as our empty bellies and looked in awe at women who had visible collarbones jutting out, thigh gaps, sharp cheekbones, and heads that looked almost alien. We dived into pro–eating disorder websites, jotting down tips and tricks for rapid and extreme weight loss. We snuck into Sophie's parents' room (we always snuck into parents' rooms FYI – if you think your young teen is not rummaging around in your drawers, you are wrong) and pulled the electric scales out from under the bed, taking turns to close our eyes as the others read out the dreaded number. We were all too thin for a while, but that wasn't the important part. Nobody wanted the highest number.

Despite all of that, for us, it wasn't simply about food or even necessarily about body image. Diet culture meant something else to me than to my mum's generation. I was shape-shifting. Working out what empty meant. How hollow felt. The *Twilight* generation, we all wanted to live between worlds, abstract, fantastical, and glittering. Concrete, static reality scared us. Look how our elders suffered! Experimenting with food was an example of us trying on an identity, letting it settle in our bodies, imagining being one of those air-brushed women. Out of focus, soft edges, blurred. We were searching for better-than-real-life, and Instagram had the answer to checking out. Adults reminded us time and time again that what we were looking at online was not actually real. We knew that. Of course we knew that. It was fakeness not thinness that drew us in. We wanted fake, an alternate universe away from reality, away from ourselves. Who wanted real life?

For whatever reason, I never became too obsessed with food in the way some of my friends did. I flirted with an eating disorder, but in my case, it never turned into a full-blown relationship. I have been vegan, vegetarian, pescatarian, dairy-free, and gluten-free, but these choices are about what is genuinely good for my body and the planet.

My mum, however, can be a bit of an Almond Mum. Her and some of her friends are Generation X, which means they have grown up trying not to 'pinch more than an inch', and her attitude to food can be weirdly toxic and, sometimes, just bizarre. I once saw her eat a single hazelnut, slowly.

'Why are you eating it like that? A single hazelnut?' I asked, watching her in horror.

She chewed it even more slowly, like a rodent, nibbling the edges intentionally, then held it up to her face. 'My favourite type of nut. Please stop eating pasta straight from the saucepan . . .'

I carried on eating my pasta and tried to ignore her, but she was in one of her hovering moods. She stood in front of the table, almost dancing, and I could tell she was about to launch into a rant, or give me some random fact, or repeat a story that I'd probably heard a million times before. But instead, she popped the hazelnut into her mouth and crunched.

'And pasta again? Can I at least add some tomatoes and cucumber?'

I looked down at my pesto pasta spoon, and opened my eyes as wide as they would go. 'You're giving Almond Mum. I don't think you're qualified to give dietary advice. And it saves washing up.'

'What's Almond Mum?'

I tell Mum about the 2013 episode of *The Real Housewives of Beverly Hills*, about Yolande Hadid with her then teenage daughter Gigi. 'Gigi told her mum that she was feeling weak after eating only half an almond, and her mum suggested having a couple of almonds and chewing them really slowly. It's a term that basically means parents who push restrictive eating habits on their kids.'

'Oof.'

'I mean, a single hazelnut . . .'

'I'm allergic to them,' she said. 'Makes my throat swell a bit.'

'You're what?! Why would you eat something you're allergic to? You're a nurse!'

'It's a mild allergy. That's why I only have one. Not about the calories.'

'So weird. OK that may not be, but remember when you gave Tay sweetcorn and peas and called them his sweets?'

'That was about protecting his teeth more than worrying about his weight.'

'That's true, but you read every single nutritional label, and you lose your mind in cereal aisles of the supermarket. You're always saying things like why not sprinkle some chia seeds on your salad? Or when we were little and begged you to go to McDonald's and you said it would kill you. That kind of thing.'

Mum laughed. 'That is true. Ultra-processed food bothers me a lot.'

'And you'd have been delighted if that microbiome test you did showed a parasite living in your gut. Let's face it.'

She laughs again. 'Delighted is a strong word, but I get your point. That's a bit messed up, isn't it?' She rubbed her throat and guzzled down a glass of water.

'I think you should just avoid hazelnuts', I said. 'As well as parasites.'

★

My contemporaries are trying to change the status quo about beauty ideals and fatness, but things are still pretty stressful for too many people. When I was younger, I remember watching the Kardashians and feeling hopeful that the ideal body image that was presented to young people for so many years was being challenged. I thought a lot about the body image consumed by us on social media being representations of not only thin but also white body types. The Kardashians offered something else in terms of body type. They were, however, pioneers of black-fishing. Cornrows on white girls and enough fake tan applied to encourage ethnic ambiguity bothered me a lot. It felt like so many celebrities were profiting from Black culture in ways that Black people are not able to. I remember following the massive trend of Brazilian butt lift surgeries being performed in overseas clinics; of watching people's recoveries – or not – posted on socials, as though the person making a video diary of their journey had climbed the Himalayas instead of using their junior ISA to have life-risking surgery for a bigger butt. Still, that felt like something better than starvation ideals. But then 'heroin chic' returned, the glamorisation of drug addiction and extreme hunger, and even the Kardashians changed shape. Shrank.

I have enough friends with eating disorders to know that sometimes food means control, and often, people want to disappear entirely. I have friends with permanent feeding tubes in their nostrils, who literally live in hospital while they try to recover. One of the saddest things is when a friend is responding to treatment, and everyone around them – teachers, parents, doctors – believes they're in recovery, but their eating disorder just has a new name. They switch online profiles from 'ED recovery' to 'gym girl', and aside from a name change, it's clear they're still struggling.

Eating disorders have changed into something new with my generation. ARFID – Avoidant/Restrictive Food Intake Disorder – is rampant. As well as avoiding entire food groups, tons of my friends will only eat beige food, or untoasted bagels, or have textural issues with food, which might be related to neurodiversity or even terror. Fear of choking is a terrifying thing to live with, and it's preventing people from eating certain things or, in some cases, eating at all. As far as I know, the link between the fear of choking leading to disordered eating and the rise in violent and misogynistic porn has not been studied. But it should be.

It's not always about fear, though; disordered eating also happens when people simply can't be bothered to eat. Maybe we're so apathetic that even eating feels like a chore.

ARFID feels like a new thing, as if it's a more socially acceptable form of dieting, but it is an eating disorder. We don't want to live in a toxic diet culture but we can't get away from the underlying issues inflicted on us by patriarchy.

Are we any better than the generations that have come before? My Grandma and her friends were obsessed with dieting, going to WeightWatchers every week and actually weighing-in in front of each other. 'Me and my friend used to not eat all day, get weighed, then go for fish and chips afterwards', she once told me. It's hard to imagine living like that.

But although Generation X, who were obsessed with celebrity magazines and thinness (whiteness) as a beauty ideal, have a healthier recognition that diet culture is toxic, pathological 'healthy eating' is on the rise in all generations. In my view this is often not about food, health, or climate, but thinness.

I dodged the bullet of a full-blown eating disorder, but I've seen too many friends lose literally years to illnesses related to food and eating. An entire life can be shaped around the culture that began with the idea that when women are smaller, it makes men feel bigger. We were lucky, both Mum and me. Things haven't really improved all that much; they are, maybe, more underground. Of course, eating disorders are often not about food at all. When you can't control absolutely anything, food is the one thing you can. Mum always says that me and my friends would have been punks in the seventies; but it feels to her like instead of anarchy we crave control, and hatred is turned inwards, not outwards. I sort of understand what she means. It's almost a miracle in our society for a young person to get through adolescence without ending up food- and body-sick.

Luckily, Mum – despite being Gen X and having weird sub-conscious ideas that lean towards being Almond Mum – had a relationship with food that was mostly about pleasure. I think throughout my childhood seeing her get excited about food in general, watching cooking shows, trying new restaurants, even planning dinner from breakfast time onwards, was help-ful. She tried to make food fun. For dessert, she'd offer us either a yoghurt or a 'Mummy special', which could be anything from ice cream with a frozen fish finger to crunched-up crisps on jelly with a pickled egg at the bottom. We always chose mummy special and encouraged any guests we had for dinner to do so, too.

Mum also seemed very happy in her own skin. A bit too happy sometimes. In her bid to make me body-positive and confident, she'd often grab her belly and do a fake belly dance around the kitchen or flash her dressing gown open and jiggle up and down, saying 'Hubba Hubba'.. No amount of therapy in the world will erase those images but I'm weirdly grateful to have a mum who, mostly, loves food, and, mostly, seems to love her body, too.

Despite seeing Mum wishing for a parasite or struggling at times with her own dieting demons, her creativity and joy in food was, for me, a powerful defence against the dark arts.

Christie

I grew up on a council estate in Stevenage during the time of SodaStream and Findus Crispy Pancakes, where my brother and I would ask the chip shop workers for scraps (the burnt bits at the bottom of the fryer) for free and the ice-cream man for broken lollies (which rendered them unsaleable). Our entire estate was a place of chicken nuggets, McDonald's as a special treat, sandwich-spread sandwiches, and no money. Everyone ate a diet consisting mainly of white bread as it was cheap, filling, and could be used alongside pretty much any meal to bulk it out, and microwavable chips. Every family home had a crisp cupboard and a chocolate box – usually an empty ice-cream box filled with three packs of Mars Bars. Nobody ever really ate out, restaurants visits were rare, and takeaway a mystical thing reserved for rich people. People ate ham sandwiches at lunch and for tea – never dinner – they had shepherd's pie or stew, all with piles more bread, and, if lucky, banana and custard for pudding. Pasta was considered exotic and, therefore, viewed with suspicion.

My house was slightly different than my friends' houses though, a source of much pain for both me and my brother, Tom. We ate dripping on toast and the usual fare of our friends at nan's house, but at home, my dad was a complete foodie – ahead of his time. He loved to cook, grew pretty much all our veggies in an allotment, and even shot much of the meat we ate (before I transitioned to vegetarianism and cheese sandwiches). While our friends were tucking into sausages and mash, we would come home to partridges or rabbits that he'd shot, dinner of a stuffed pig's heart with home-grown marrow. We would be horrified washing mud off our apples, asking why we couldn't have them wrapped in plastic like everyone else. My mum was never as much of a food person as my dad, but she tried to keep up. Once she announced that she'd make a French bouillabaisse, much to our collective disgust; I remember both me and my brother groaning and asking for chicken dippers and oven chips. But she insisted, went off to the fishmonger that morning, and spent a fortune we most likely didn't have, only to make a dinner that resembled grey dishwater. After trying one mouthful, we ate beans on toast instead, a meal we finally appreciated. I look back with shame at my lack of appreciation for the food in our house. We were so lucky. We had no idea that food was about so much more than just that. It was story. Heritage. History. It gave my dad joy and purpose, and despite having no money growing up, he made sure we ate like kings.

Even then, growing up in a foodie environment, in a time before social media, I ended up weird about food and too conscious of my weight. When I was Rowan's age, and pretty much all through my late teenage years, I tried every diet. I remember doing the Cabbage Soup Diet, Atkins, Caveman, Ayurvedic, WeightWatchers, juice cleanse, detox, plant-based, fruitarian, Special K. For a number of years, I had a Post-it stuck to my fridge with a Kate Moss quote: 'Nothing tastes as good as skinny feels.'[6]

The Cabbage Soup Diet had my dad opening every single window and swearing loudly about the stench coming from the cabbages or perhaps from my own body, since I'd eaten so many cabbages. It was short-lived. I was always pretty skinny as a teenager, and the diets didn't really do much; partly, I suspect, as they were impossible to maintain in any case, and also my sixteen-year-old metabolism could manage the dramatic changes in my food intake without yo-yoing.

I moved in with my nan for a while when I was fifteen or sixteen. She was doing the SlimFast diet at the time, so I joined her, despite already being whip-thin. I lost a stack of much-needed weight, but she kept putting more and more on. I wondered at first if it was the one meal that we were eating in the evening, as my nan – an ex-school cook and Welsh – slathered everything in lard. But it transpired that she was having breakfast, lunch, and dinner as well as two SlimFast meal shakes.

'These are meal replacements', I told her, holding up a strawberry milkshake that smelled like vomit. 'You skip breakfast and lunch and have a shake instead, then a normal meal in the evening.'

My nan looked at me in horror. 'You mean it replaces food? Doesn't cancel out the calories?'

I nodded. 'It's not to have *with* food. *Instead of* food.'

She took the milkshake out of my hand and tipped it down the sink. 'Ridiculous', she said. 'No wonder I'm putting on weight.'

I began my nursing training in mental health, working in various hospital and community settings, and looked after many young children and adolescents as well as adults, with eating disorders. When I transferred to paediatrics from mental health nursing and moved to work at Great Ormond Street Hospital, I was surprised to find that food and eating was a significant cause of distress for many children and families, whether people had a diagnosed mental illness or not. I cared for adolescents who were hospitalised with obesity and on 'fat reducing diets', children who were literally monitored and watched on the ward twenty-four hours a day but still, somehow, managed to sneak in a burger. I worked the odd shift on the hospital inpatient unit for children experiencing a wide range of mental health issues, including eating disorders. My job as a very inexperienced student nurse was to sit and eat lunch with the young people, normalise food and joy and conversation at the dinner table. It was often excruciating. I remember one girl who would eat tiny amounts of food, cut up very small, chewing so many times, who would then beg to go to the bathroom. The toilets were locked post lunch to prevent 'purging', and although I could see the logic in terms of keeping people safe, I felt like a prison warden telling a young person only a few years younger than I was that she couldn't pee until the toilets were opened again in an hour. I remember it all feeling so desperate. While she waited for the toilet to open, the girl struggling with anorexia would flick through magazines with dozens and dozens of images of air-brushed, unattainable, skinny bodies of supposedly grown women.

Times have changed and things have moved on beyond belief in terms of body positivity and recognising that the diet culture of my generation was astonishingly toxic. But still, despite Rowan and her friends growing up in this more accepting age, many Gen X people have inevitably passed on capitalist ideals and personal neuroses. Of course, I tried not to voice any subconscious, self-destructive, deep-rooted anxieties about my body to Rowan, pretty standard fare for anyone woman who grew up when I did; but, inevitably, she absorbed everything, and having a Gen X mum, combined with social media and dance school her whole life, surely put her at high risk of disordered eating. Regardless of living in this age of anti-shaming in all forms, many of her friends had eating disorders, dancers or not. For a few years, Rowan attended an all-girls school in an affluent area, a school I'd assumed based on Ofsted analysis would be inclusive with excellent pastoral care; yet, Ro described it as horrific: 'Try going to the loos at lunchtime, you can't pee as there's a queue of pukers, and roll up anyone's shirtsleeves, you'll see how functional and high-achieving those girls are.' She went on to tell me that she knew only one person who didn't have disordered eating in some form.

Things haven't moved on as far as I imagined they would. For many young people, they are worse.

The Children's Commissioner (1st August 2023) reported that NHS figures show a large and recent increase, almost doubling in less than a decade, in the numbers of hospital admissions for young people due to eating disorders.[7] The *Guardian* reported that 1.25 million Britons have an eating disorder.[8] In November 2023, the NHS found one in eight people aged seventeen to nineteen had an eating disorder the previous year, with four times as many young women as young men making up the numbers.[9] I have a friend whose daughter has been close to death on many occasions struggling with anorexia. She does not think her daughter will make it to adulthood, and the devastating, terrifying truth is that she might be right: The National Institute of Health and Care Excellence (NICE) reports that anorexia nervosa has a higher mortality rate than any other mental health disorder and 20 per cent of those deaths are from suicide.[10]

There have been times when I've worried about Rowan's eating and times when she's been worried about mine. Conversations between us around food and diet culture were never easy and often confrontational. When Rowan told me that friends of hers were throwing up in the school toilets after lunch, I would listen whenever she went to the bathroom and stare at her knuckles for the telltale signs of bulimia. If she pushed food around her plate or told me she wasn't hungry, my insides would fill up with anxiety. I was hypervigilant for other warning signs, too. I knew that rituals, for example, using only certain kinds of crockery, chewing food very slowly, or cutting food into tiny pieces or uniform portion sizes, might be a cause for worry. When Ro would only sit in one chair at mealtimes, my radar was up. I watched out for other early warning signs, but they were almost impossible to separate from the Gen Z zeitgeist – tracking of steps, using a Fitbit, removing entire food groups from a diet, increased interest in health. Some symptoms of an eating disorder, I thought, might apply to all teenagers and be signs of adolescence: low body confidence, fluctuations in mood, and deception (I already ate, I'm not hungry, I'm having dinner at so-and-so's house).

I watched like a hawk and tried to pretend I was totally casual about eating and my body. It was not easy. But I tried really hard to enjoy food around Ro, and in our house, we always tried to avoid triggering words. We talked at length about the gift that nursing gives, of appreciating bodies that simply work. Being able-bodied and to move, dance, breathe, eat, laugh, walk, and run are not things I ever take for granted.

Of course, I have so much work still to do, to accept and love my body completely and every day, and try and be a better role model for Ro. Despite my best efforts, I felt a flicker of disappointment when my Zoe test results came back, and I did not have the parasite after all.

Christie's Fridge

Olives; Gouda; Manchego; Pickles; Chutneys; Peppers; Tomatoes; Cucumber; Spring onions; Red onions; Shallots; Broccoli; Cavolo Nero; Organic chicken; Almond milk (unsweetened); Kimchi; Salmon; Dark chocolate; Coconut water; White wine; Lamb's lettuce; Radishes.

Ro's Fridge

Four packets of Value Feta; Vitamin C.

CONVERSATIONS

PATRIARCHY

Christie: Do you want to hold her? She's ready for a feed, so it doesn't matter if she wakes.

Paternal Grandpa: Yes. My grandbaby! I've been waiting so long for my grandchild to be born.

Christie: Her name is Bella.

Paternal Grandfather: Her name is Kikelomo.

Christie: We can use that as her middle name. It's very beautiful.

Paternal Grandpa: She is Kikelomo. And now you are MamaKike. In Nigeria, when the first child is born, the mother changes her name. You are born, too.

Christie: I love that. Does the father also change their name?

Paternal Grandpa: Hahaha, no. Only mummy.

Christie: Hmmm.

Paternal Grandma: A girl.

Christie: A daughter. We're so happy.

Paternal Grandpa: Don't worry. Next one will be a boy.

Christie: *Silence.*

BOOMERS

Maternal Grandma: How's Bella? I miss her so much. Hope she's doing a bit better?

Christie: Bella is now Rowan . . .

Maternal Grandma: What do you mean?

Christie: She's changing her name. Rowan.

Maternal Grandma: *Silence.*

Christie: She doesn't want a gendered name.

Maternal Grandma: Ridiculous.

Christie: I feel a bit sad about it. I chose that name and love it so much.

Maternal Grandma: Ridiculous.

Christie: It could be worse. Rowan is not bad.

Maternal Grandma: Ridiculous.

Christie: *Silence.*

Maternal Grandma: I won't be calling her that. I'll be calling her Bella. She's Bella. She can call herself what she likes but people will just call her Bella.

Christie: She's changed her name at school. They all call her Rowan. Legally, she can change her name officially now, though she hasn't mentioned that yet.

Maternal Grandma: Well, the school can't call her Rowan without your permission . . .

Christie: They can. They do.

Maternal Grandma: That's not right. Ridiculous.

Christie: I love the name Bella. But it is gendered. If she feels non-binary, maybe she has a point.

Maternal Grandma: *Long silence.*

THE SILENT GENERATION
(A FEW WEEKS LATER)

Maternal Grandma: She's called Rowan now.

Great Grandma: What, love?

Maternal Grandma: Bella. She goes by Rowan.

Great Grandma: I don't understand. Did you read in the *Mirror* about that woman in Scotland? Waited fourteen hours for an ambulance. Terrible state it's in, our country.

Maternal Grandma: Bella is changing her name. To Rowan. It was too gendered.

Great Grandma: What do you mean, love? Bella is both her great-great-grandmothers' names, Isabella. That's why she's called Bella. After her great-great-grandmothers.

Maternal Grandma: Well, she goes by Rowan now.

Great Grandmother: I'll call her Bella. I don't understand. You mean Bella?

Maternal Grandma: It's just a name. Rowan suits her, actually. It was a shock for me, too, at first, but it's just a name. It's hard to understand, I know. Point is, she's doing really well at the moment. I think Rowan is quite lovely really.

Great Grandmother. *Silence.*

CHAPTER FOUR

Sugar and Spice and All Things Nice

Gender

Rowan: My friend forgot his binder, can you see if it's in the wash? He can't find it and I think he might have left it on my bedroom floor.

Christie: What's a binder? Also, you do know that there is no magic washing fairy, right?

Rowan: It's to help trans people. I did a load of washing on Tuesday.

Christie: Ro, it's now Sunday. And please don't just chuck in everything if you've only worn it once and it's clean. Your jeans were in there this morning, and I only washed them two days ago.

Rowan: It's really tight.

Christie: Sounds a bit like my sports bra . . .

Rowan: Kai hates people calling it that.

Christie: *Pause. A beat.* Why did you have your friend's binder?

Rowan: When Kai stayed over, he left it by accident. He's got a spare but he needs it.

Christie: How long do you wear them for? It's probably still on your bedroom floor along with everything else in the universe.

Rowan: Six hours max. Under eighteen.

Christie: I know, I know, my sports bra is not the same, but it really is too tight. In fact, I might go to Marks & Spencer later if you want to come and get a new one. Oh! We could have pancakes in Brixton market. We haven't had lunch out together for ages.

Rowan: *Glares.* Mum, you need to stop with the sports bra thing. And no, I never want to go to Marks & Spencer.

Christie: Is there any correlation between binders and corsets?

Rowan: *Slightly confused silence.*

Christie: Hang on, who is Kai? Do they identify as a boy? And why did you have a boy staying in your bedroom?

Rowan: *Rolls eyes.* Kai used to be called Annabel.

Christie: Annabel identifies as a boy now?

Rowan: *Rolls eyes and head.* No. Kai is a boy.

Christie: If Annabel is now Kai, *he* shouldn't be sharing a bed with you. You're fifteen years old.

Rowan: Mum, Kai is gay.

Christie: *Slightly confused silence.* I don't understand but I'm trying.

Rowan: Try harder.

Christie

When I was fifteen, I wore DM boots and oversized jumpers found exclusively in charity shops and spent hours in Stevenage town centre giving out leaflets of rabbits with red bleeding eyes urging people not to wear cosmetics. I wore a badge that said 'Fuck Off', smoked roll-ups and stayed out hours past my curfew with a Black Sabbath tribute band. But it was only when I shaved my head that my dad sat me down to 'have a chat'. He was worried about me, he said. I remember him shaking a bit, which was extremely unusual. It made me nervous. Perhaps they were getting a divorce? They'd been arguing a bit. Maybe I'd have to live a week at a time with each parent moving between houses like my friend Sharon, who said her life was like a depressingly slow and tragic game of ping pong, and she was the ball. Perhaps – like Sharon – we would not be able to afford to stay in town and would have to move to the country-side or face other fates worse than death. Of course, my dramatic teenage brain did not consider even once that the cause of their stress might, in fact, be parenting me.

'Do you have anything to tell me?' My dad smiled the most uncomfortable smile I'd ever seen and loosely draped his arm on my shoulder. It has been thirty years since that conversation and I can still remember the coldness of his arm, the smell of his T-shirt, the feeling of doom in my stomach. 'If you're gay, you can tell us, you know.'

A few seconds. I heard ticking but there was no clock in the room. Then I laughed a bit. He looked as confused as I felt and a little hurt. 'We will understand. Totally accept it. It will mean life is hard, at times, I imagine. But of course, we'll understand.'

I looked at my dad's face. He was searching. Not for clues about my sexuality but something else. Trying to solve a difficult problem, like I was algebra. Of course, he didn't understand. Him and my mum had no idea about anything. Something separated us, a generational gap that was invisible to the outside eye but not to us.

I shook off his arm, a bit angry by then. That's how quickly my moods shifted. The nervous, relieved laughter evaporated and instead I was left hot in the middle, with hormones like molten lava, my teenage volcano-brain ready to blow. 'What do you mean life will be hard? I mean, what are you talking about? It shouldn't matter who people love. Why is it anyone's business?'

I could see my dad sink into his suspicions, visibly deflate. He was pretty progressive, and yet, here he was worried about what the world would be like for me. Nowadays I realise how lucky I was, and how many of my queer friends would have appreciated my dad's understanding. So many people are assaulted, made homeless, and ostracised from families for all kinds of reasons when coming out. But I did not appreciate my dad's careful concern. We were sitting so close together, but I could see the distance between us. For the first time, there was a wide gap, and he was far, far away from me.

'Why is life harder for gay people? I'll tell you why. Because people of your generation are so homophobic. Dinosaurs!' I knew my dad wasn't intentionally homophobic and I could see his hurt eyes but I couldn't stop. I ranted and ranted about homophobia and how his generation could never understand mine and how the world was totally different to when he was young. And then later, after I snuck out with the Black Sabbath tribute band, I cried tears of anger and, of course, guilt. I cried on the shoulder of my boyfriend – as it happens. 'I wish I was gay', I said.

When Rowan was fifteen, it was a very confusing time. A steady stream of adolescents descended on my daughter's bedroom and occasionally came out for vegan or dairy-free or gluten-free meals. But sleepovers were no longer simply about ordering pizza and putting in earplugs: I had awkward phone-calls with parents of teens about whether sharing a bed was a dangerous act. I didn't ask if her friend is a boy or girl, as Rowan said that kind of question was extremely offensive, and besides, she scoffed, assumes that there are only *two* genders. 'You can ask about identity but not boy/girl. Half my friends are neither', she told me. Asking about friends' gender was off the table and sexuality was 'absolutely none of my business'. *I don't ask your friends what they have in their pants or do in their bedrooms.*

It was a fair point, but how do we parents then manage risk? In the old days, the rules seemed easy. Heteronormative as it was, a boyfriend would simply not be allowed to share a bed with a fifteen-year-old daughter. But who was a boyfriend now? What is gender? What is sexuality? What does daughter mean? We parents discussed impending sleepovers on the phone, and I explained that Rowan has proposed their child share her bedroom and asked how they feel about it. Responses ranged from 'that's fine, he's very gay' to 'they are asexual, so I think it's OK'. Then there was a pause and some sadness underneath the words.

I understood the sadness. I could still feel the cold skin of my dad's arm on my shoulder. Rowan imagined that sadness comes from a place of non-acceptance, just as I did all those years ago. But I heard my dad's voice echo inside mine as though words are footprints we walk in. The world is not easy in the margins. Sometimes it is not even safe. I wanted Rowan to be exactly herself, to find out who she was and (in the words of Dolly Parton) 'do it on purpose'. But she still had much to learn. And so did I.

I have always had LGBTQIA+ friends ('Most of your friends are gay', Ro often reminded me), as well as disabled friends, from many diverse cultures and backgrounds. But even with many friends of marginalised identities, who have shaped, changed and influenced my thinking, mothering in this political climate is sometimes really difficult. When Rowan changed her name from Bella, one of the reasons she gave was that it was too gendered. In the next breath she announced that she did not believe that gender exists at all. 'Call me she/her/they/them or he/him', she said. 'It really doesn't matter. Preferably just Rowan. I'll change it officially. Bella is too feminine.'

When I challenged her that if gender did not exist, or at least should not exist, which is what I think she was getting at, then how could the name Bella be too gendered?

It was confusing. But I tried to listen. I listened to Rowan and her friends and their inclusive language and acceptance. I listened to an older friend (and other gender-critical second-wave feminist friends) who feared that 'woman' has become a dirty word and that the fighting they've done their whole life was being undone. I listened to my friend, a trans man, who was wounded every time he was misgendered and suffered so much transphobic abuse. I listened to a midwife friend who refused to use the terms suggested by NHS guidelines for trans and non-binary patients like 'pregnant person' as opposed to 'woman', 'chest-feeding' as opposed to 'breastfeeding', and another midwife friend who believed inclusive language to be an essential part of quality care.

It was not even that there were two camps but many and so many voices, all either shouting or being silenced. These arguments and sometimes toxic attitudes in all directions were perhaps an expression of collective pain. There must be a way through. I know many parents who are struggling to understand their child's gender or sexual identity and who feel a bit lost or, at least, left behind. Cultural change is always a time of anxiety, but it's also a beautiful time. Generation Z are building on the LGBTQIA+ activists of previous generations to try and make ours a fairer society. 'It's not that deep', Ro told me.

'Doesn't have to be complicated.' She attended a dance conservatoire where the teens could no longer be separated or split into genders.

'There are many young people in the class who don't identify with boy or girl', the teacher said. 'And how they identify might change next week. Everyone is fluid.'

But the solution – to split roles according to who wanted to do what – was astonishingly simple.

Other parts of our country might not have such a progressive attitude. I could only imagine the conversations in leadership teams of single sex schools. Teachers, I did not envy.

But parents, I think, must learn, and try to understand the very real struggles of young people living in the margins. It is our job to try to keep our children safe and part of that means examining structural and individual biases and prejudices about sexuality and gender. Books are helpful. Podcasts. Avoiding echo chambers and actively seeking conversations with people of different ages and who have differing viewpoints is useful. Nuance is essential. We can foster an inclusive space for everyone while also acknowledging some difficult truths. Two facts can be true at once:

The world is too often an unsafe place for all women.

The world is too often an unsafe place for trans people.

Change happens when we are all less binary. Half the time, when I hear people arguing, I wonder if people are fighting for exactly the same core thing: safety and freedom in a patriarchal society. We are all so human. All of us. Desperately fragile, complex, tricky, flawed humans. Each and every one of us is connected and has so much in common. During this time of great division, between right- and left-wing politics and old and younger generations, it is this raw humanity that binds us. It's in the space when we disagree, respectfully, that real political and cultural change exists. There is no us and them in any sense. Just us and us. We all deserve to live without violence and targeted abuse. We all deserve safety and love. We are all so vulnerable and complicated, and for each and every one of us, our lives can turn on a dime. The only thing that matters really is kindness, and not performative kindness we might see on a banner or an Instagram post, but real-to-the-core kindness that most of us are lucky to have witnessed in our lives. Often from strangers. Sometimes from people we might fundamentally disagree with. Being a mum – and being a daughter – is learning that you can clash on many things and still love each other anyway. We all can.

Rowan

'I'm changing my name', I told Mum. She was sitting in the living room, reading a newspaper and watching the news at the same time, which seemed like overkill. She didn't look at me, so I hovered in the doorway. I wasn't scared, exactly, but it was good to have an escape route if she started to shout. Spies are great at exit strategies, and so are teenagers. 'I'm called Rowan now. Not Bella.'

This time, she looked at me. 'What are you talking about?'

'Bella is too gendered. I'm going to be Rowan. From now on. When I'm sixteen, I'll change it legally, by deed poll. I've looked it up. I can do that.'

'You can't just do whatever you want in life, you know. If Bella is too gendered, and you don't believe in gender, that makes no sense.'

I felt my blood boiling a bit, which it always did when Mum didn't listen properly. But I didn't want an argument. I didn't know how to respond to her. I know how I felt and why I want to change my name. But I hadn't rehearsed a comeback.

'Bella is a beautiful name', she went on. And on and on. 'It suits you. And it's a lovely name.'

'Rowan suits me better', I said and stomped upstairs.

In the safety of my bedroom, I carried on the conversation with her, to the air. I told her that even though I don't believe in gender, everyone else still does. We live in a totally gendered society. If my name is Bella, they immediately assume feminine, girly, *beautiful*; that's how people see and treat me. I whisper-reminded Mum (who was still downstairs) of when we went to Italy when I was a toddler, and how everyone shouted Bella, Bellisima, Bella Bambino, to the extent I got whiplash thinking people were calling *me*, rather than just commenting that I was a cute baby girl. A generic beautiful cutesy baby who everyone felt ownership towards and could project onto. I didn't want to be a cute anything. I didn't want to be a girl. I didn't want to be a boy either. I think gender is a bullshit concept. I am Rowan. Just a person. A human.

One of my earliest memories is Kai telling me he wanted to be a boy. We were five years old, and back then he was known as Annabelle. Later that year, he said he didn't mean it. And he looked very sad after that. He stopped laughing. He stopped talking. He shrank. When Kai turned fifteen, he came out to his parents. He explained that his gender identity doesn't align with his biological sex, and it feels like living outside himself and looking down on someone else the entire time. Kai's parents did not take it well. They refused to call him by his name. They said it was fashionable and that his friends were influencing him to be trans. They were afraid, I guess. They said life would be so hard for him if he chose to live that way. But life is hard for him already. Kai has a pet dog, a small Jack Russell called Ziggy, who he used to walk every day. Honestly, I can't tell you how much he loves that dog. He's now so uncomfortable in the way he looks and feels that he won't leave his house, not even to walk Ziggy. He's in pain in so many different ways. His back aches due to continuously forcing bad posture on himself in an attempt to conceal his body. Whenever possible, he'll avoid showering, not because he's just a teenage boy that doesn't like to wash but because it would mean he'd have to see himself in the mirror and it'd be someone else staring back. A stranger. Imagine not recognising yourself in the mirror.

He knows who he is though. He has always known since we were five years old. Life is hard for him not because of who he is but because society doesn't accept him, and that starts at home; his parents do not see who he is. They only see the reflection that he doesn't recognise. They don't understand at all. He is not choosing this. The only choice here is theirs. Why can't they listen? Where is the intervention from other adults? How hard is it to call a person by their name?

Kai went to a different secondary school to mine, but I know he stopped doing any work. He had wanted to be an architect. Now he stays in bed all day. His dad took away his binder. His mum walks the dog.

As teenagers, my friends and I almost never discussed each other's gender. It was not a thing. To me and my friends, it was meaningless. We tended to accept how someone wanted to identify. That's it. It's really not that difficult. Ask someone who they are, and they will tell you. But to some of my friends' parents, and so many people in older generations, it feels like the issue of our time. I think climate change, war, AI, the threats to democracy, and the destruction of our planet are more pressing issues, but there you go.

Maybe it's politically convenient to divide and conquer while all these bigger things are going on. Make people hate each other. Make older people hate younger people. Make everyone hate the trans community (who, in my experience, are the sweetest people alive, who've had the most struggles). Of course, we've all experienced discrimination of one sort or another, but my trans friends have really been through it. I wonder if transphobia is because we are in the process of a sea change. My generation are continuing a decades- (even century-) long fight to deconstruct gender itself, and it's destabilising.. Change is necessary, and it is happening, whether people like it or not. But it feels so dangerous right now for people outside gender norms. It's pretty shocking that we're seeing a culture-war backlash like never before, despite the huge leaps that the generations before ours have made for LGBTQIA+ rights.

At the time of writing, it has now been a year since Brianna

Ghey was stabbed twenty-eight times in the back in Cheshire, in a murder fuelled by sadism and transphobia. On 8 February 2024, Nex Benedict, a two spirit, transgender, and gender non-conforming sixteen-year-old died after what has so far only been described as a 'physical altercation' in their high school bathroom in Oklahoma. On 13 February 2024 in Harrow, London, a trans girl was stabbed fourteen times at a roller-skating party. How many more young people must die?

Surely, we need to make institutions like hospitals and schools and communities much safer for trans – and all – people. We need to find a way to talk about gender without shouting. A toxic debate only serves politicians, not regular people. A more accepting world can only be a good thing for everyone.

'Shall I order a pizza?' Mum was sitting on the couch opposite and trying to be chirpy. She was happy that I was home and that my friend and I were downstairs instead of in my bedroom. My friend, Frankie, was new to my school, and it was the first time they'd been over. I could see they were nervous about meeting Mum, and a bit shy. Mum smiled. 'By the way, Frankie, what pronouns do you prefer? As well as what pizza toppings?'

Frankie flicked their head up. They were not used to that. 'They them. Thank you for asking.'

'You're very welcome', Mum said. 'Any preference for pizza toppings?'

'Vegetarian', I said, 'extra chilli.'

Frankie nodded. Mum got up to go find her phone, and as soon as she was out of earshot, Frankie whispered to me. 'Your mum is actually lovely.'

'It shouldn't be lovely to ask someone's pronouns, just normal.'

'I was talking about the pizza', Frankie said, and we both started laughing.

CONVERSATIONS

CAPITALISM

Rowan: I'm going to live off grid.

Christie: What are you talking about?

Rowan: Off grid. That's what I'm planning.

Christie: What does 'off' grid mean? By the way, did you write Aunty Gill a thank you for your birthday voucher?

Rowan: I'll avoid capitalist ideals. Live off the land. Get a small-holding. I don't want to be owned by the state.

Christie: Honestly, Rowan, I don't know what you're talking about. You're saying you don't want to work?

Rowan: Your generation work too much. To pay for shit you don't need or want with money you don't actually have. It's a total scam.

Christie: Agree. But not about work. I love my work.

Rowan: You work all the time. At what cost . . .

Christie: I do. I know, I know. But OK, as you appear to have retired before even day one of a working life, how will you support yourself?

Rowan: I told you. I'll live off the land.

Christie: You couldn't even keep a plant alive. Not even cacti.

Rowan: *Short silence.*

Christie: It's good to work. If you find a job you love, you'll never work a day in your life.

Rowan: Or you could just never work a day in your life. I basically want to lie in bed and read all day. That's my plan. I just want peace. Freedom.

Christie: Good for you. I feel the same.

Rowan: Slay.

CHAPTER FIVE

Chicken Nugget Face

Social Media

Christie: (with Snapchat photo filter of her face as an apple): How do you like them apples?

Rowan:

Rowan

There's no need to see white before red. It's a phrase people use to mean 'don't take things too far'. It stems from a self-harm situation gone wrong, when you've cut deep and gone to the bone. When I told Mum this, she looked faint and had to put her head between her legs and take deep breaths. She was pretty squeamish for an ex-nurse.

'I didn't have a single friend who was self-harming', she told me. 'Not in that way. Not when I was at school.'

She called a few friends, all women roughly the same age of around mid- to late-forties, and they all concurred. Nobody in their friendship group was cutting. Nobody was burning themselves, or picking skin off, or pulling hair and eyelashes out. Nobody. It's not that mental health wasn't a problem. They had eating disorders and depression and anxiety, but not to the extent that young people do now, not by a long, long way. Self-harm was not a thing.

That fact astonished me. I knew tons of girls who started cutting their arms at twelve years old. Tons. I was a bit tempted at that age, but something stopped me, despite wanting to experience the relief it seemed to offer them. But then, I was the oldest in my friend group to get a smartphone. I don't think that is a coincidence. My mum refused to give me access to a phone and social media until I was fourteen, which is still young, but it was two years after my friends. Even then, at first, she monitored my phone – the condition of having one was that at any random moment she'd do a 'phone check', and I would hand the phone over to her without question. She'd check that there wasn't anything dangerous. She was wild eyed and worried but never found anything more than gossip about teachers, once a chat about a racist teacher who a friend described as the kind of person who masturbated to *Roots*.

But Mum had no idea what she was looking for. We spoke a different language. She struggled with the TV remote, let alone smartphone tech, apps, and the dark web. I was never big on Instagram and didn't go near Twitter or Facebook, which felt like a forum for older people (if my grandma was on it, it was probably not my thing). But TikTok stole a few years of my life, no doubt, and WhatsApp and Snapchat groups gave that time a dark texture, for sure.

I had secretly joined a group chat that Mum did not know about, which was akin to an online psych ward. The group changed me, though I'm not sure if it was helpful or damaging. Maybe, like all social media, it was both things. We'd all stay up chatting to each other until 6 a.m., before falling asleep and doing it all again the next day. If I was away from the chat for even five minutes, I'd have hundreds of notifications. For around eight months during the final year of lockdowns, we chatted online constantly, addictively, to the exclusion of real life. There was no real life going on anyway. I guess it was a form of brainwashing that affected us the most. Constant communication and no escape.

All of us had mental health issues, posting pictures or videos of self-harm, and mental illness became a competitive sport. We spent much of our time messaging, trying to stop each other from hurting or killing ourselves; but looking back, I wonder if we were doing the opposite. I don't know how many messages I've sent to friends, or received from friends, trying to convince them to 'not do anything stupid'. It's wild to me now. It was a full-time job for a while, trying to keep my friends alive via WhatsApp messaging groups. Trying to stay alive myself.

The more I tried to constantly communicate with friends in that forum, the further away Mum seemed to be. There was a good chunk of time when she didn't seem to know how to communicate with me at all. I knew little about her life and she knew little about mine. We could be literally sitting next to each other, yet it felt like we were on the other side of the world. She'd ask me a question, repeat it, then frame exactly the same question in a different way; so our chats were at first stilted and boring, then annoying. I stopped listening. She stopped asking.

The first time she sent me a Snapchat-filtered photo of her, her head was a piece of broccoli. She had added a Dr Dre sound-track in the background and written, *New Year New Me*. At that moment, I thought she had actually lost it. Nothing about Mum made any sense to me, but somehow this did. Despite being so angry with her for pretty much everything, I looked at the photo for a long time, and I remember thinking that we would be OK. I have no idea why I thought that. She was clearly unhinged. But something made me message back: a laughing face. This spurred her on. The only way I'd commu-nicate with her was if she sent me a stupid meme or Snapchat version of her face as a horse or packet of chips or some-thing. Sometimes she'd write little quotes to go with the photo, *Missing you*, or *Like my lashes?* Or *How do you like them apples?* Once, she sent a photo of her with massive thick dark eye-brows, and wrote, *Are my eyebrows en fleek?* She was trying to speak my language, and sometimes it made me laugh, other times was just cringy. But all of a sudden, after not talking at all, there were dozens of photos of her on my phone, disguised as food, but her eyes staring at me. Mum as a dumpling, the words: *You'll always be my little dumpling*. Her and my brother as bears, with: *Look for the bear necessities*. Mum as a bird of prey: *Fly High Bruh*. Always a Prince or Madonna or Gangster Rap soundtrack. I have no idea what it was about this that made me respond despite vowing silence towards her. The silliness of it, maybe. There was something about her randomness, and her acceptance of that, which made me feel better about her, and about me. It felt like she would always try and find me, wherever I was and whatever it took. There was humour to be found even in dreadful places. There is power in that. It was hard to think suicidal thoughts when looking at Mum disguised as a dumpling.

Every now and then she'd try and use actual words, to tell me something interesting she'd done that day; to be fair, she did lead an interesting life, but even then, I zoned out and couldn't wait to get away and talk to my friends. Mealtimes were brutal, particularly Sundays. She'd spend hours cooking a roast dinner, then call me and my brother, the two of us eating with our heads down, racing through the meal so we could get back to whatever we were doing. Mum would chew each mouthful slowly, try to strike up conversations, asking us about friends or school, or in my case, dance. When we shrugged or gave one-word answers, she'd get upset and point out that it is nice to talk and share a meal and that she'd been cooking for hours. I would remind her that we didn't ask her to do that, cook a roast dinner, and we didn't ask to be born. Mum then got even more upset, and the Sunday vibe would descend, sometimes ending in silence and other times in shouting. You never knew what you'd get on Sundays: chicken or beef, silence or shouting.

We weren't alone in our lack of ability to communicate effectively with each other. At that time, pretty much none of my friends were speaking to their parents. Not in any real sense. There didn't seem to be any need to talk to them, who felt oceans apart from us; there was no point in small talk. Mum and I went from discussing everything, all the time, to a black hole of nothingness. But we found a way back from it with stupid filters. I don't know if that was time, or silly fun, or my mental health improving, or growing up a bit. But I think it was mostly about Mum hanging in there. Knowing she would always speak to me, whenever I was ready, in any way I'd listen, helped a lot. That she never gave up trying to communicate with me. Even when I was a raging arsehole. Even when she was.

Christie

Come home urgently. I need you to film me in a bathtub full of frozen peas.

Rowan had not spoken to me for a week or so by this point. We were in our non-communication phase. Still, this text elicited an immediate response. Perhaps it was the urgency of it, or maybe the strangeness. In any case, she text. *K.*

I rushed to the supermarket and filled up the trolley with bag after bag of frozen peas. The cashier frowned but said nothing as she scanned twenty-five bags in total. But she muttered something inaudible as I walked away. It must have seemed so odd, my behaviour. It was odd. But it was all I had. My dear friend's husband had just died, and we had history with peas.

I first met Jess while researching another book. An old-school nurse working in the justice system, she was tough and compassionate and no nonsense and as stoic as nurses come. But life had tested all of that. Her husband had suffered with cancer for years, and they'd had to navigate the worst of all things. She had expected that when he died, although devastating, it would be a sort of relief in any case. A door opening to recovery, or the possibility of it. But the shock of it was shocking. Even when inevitable. She called me, choking on words; she sounded as if she was drowning in oil. The pain unbearable. I didn't know what to say.

Jess always knew what to do and what to say though, even when words were not enough. When Rowan was seriously ill, and I'd phoned her in the night unable to speak as I was crying too hard, she had simply been there on the other end of the phone. Later, she sent me a short video of herself in her mother's disabled bath, eating a bowlful of peas with a giant spoon. It had made absolutely no sense at all, yet broke through something and despite all of it, had made me laugh. Laughter is healing. Briefly, humour can light up even the darkest of times. Every nurse knows this. And Rowan knows it, too.

I filled the bath, emptying in the peas one bag after the other until the bath was full. 'I'll put a swimsuit on.'

'I'd appreciate that', Ro said. But she didn't mention the peas. She had no questions.

I came back into the bathroom, holding a large serving spoon, and climbed into the pea bath. 'Jess's husband died', I said. Rowan hadn't asked for an explanation. But I felt the need to explain in any case. 'I have no idea what it means, doing this, but I know somehow that she'll appreciate it. It will break through something, however briefly.'

Rowan took out her phone and began preparing the shot. 'You don't need to explain.'

She filmed me in the bath, eating the peas with a giant spoon, and I later sent the clip to Jess, writing: *No words. Just peas.* Random, bizarre humour always helps me, and Jess, even in our darkest hours. A flash of connection between me and Jess, and between me and Rowan.

For around a year after that, our communication was terrible. Rowan barely spoke to me at all. She wouldn't answer the phone, or texts, and in person simply grunted. I tried writing letters. Sending bright and breezy notes. I tried keeping my cool. But after radio silence, I inevitably lost it fairly frequently and ended up shouting, or sending long rambling messages about respect and politeness, or angry Post-it notes. Nothing seemed to have any effect. It was like living with a stranger.

Eventually, I remembered her responding to the peas, her love of the random, her odd humour. I opened Snapchat and scrolled through to find the most ridiculous filters. One that turned my face into a chicken nugget, another that made me morph into a piece of sushi. I would click on the image and send it off to Rowan. Nine times out of ten, despite not really speaking to me at that time, she would respond almost immediately. I sent her my face as an apple, and the line underneath: *How do you like them apples?* She sent back a laughing face. I sent me disguised as a chip, or a horse, or a chipmunk. She responded every time, and each reply made my heart sing a little. A crumb of communication. A morsel of connection, aided by my degradation. Humour and stupidity helped us find each other in the darkness. Social media offered us a space to communicate in new ways.

But, of course, social media was not always helpful.

Smartphones could be as harmful to children as smoking and gambling, reported Devi Sridhar in the *Guardian*.[11] The grassroots movement Smartphone Free Childhood, report that 97 per cent of twelve-year-olds in Britain have a smartphone. The research is overwhelming: Smartphones expose children to harmful content, raise the likelihood of developing a mental illness, and are highly addictive.

It's strange to me now imagining the teenage landscape that I grew up in, on the whole, devoid of dangers that teens now face thanks to technology: self-harm, sexting and nudes, cyber bullying, easy access to (violent) porn. I can't conceive of how it must feel for an argument at school, rumours, gossip, even violence to follow you home and continue all night. The notion of keeping a child safely at home, in their bedrooms, is redundant. I was a teen in the nineties, and we had real-life flashers, a phenomenon that is baffling to Rowan. Because sexual predators are now online, operating virtually. Our children carry them around in their pockets.

The US Surgeon General Dr Vivek Murthy issued an advisory about the effects of social media on youth mental health, stating, 'There is growing evidence that social media use is associated with harm to young people's mental health.'[12] If you Google (ironically perhaps) social media mental health, there's a ton of research and articles, some of them contradictory, but most linking a rise in adolescent mental illness to the use of social media. My psychiatrist and psychologist friends tell me that it is one of the biggest contributing factors to mental illness in teens. The Priory Group website and *The Washington Post* report some shocking statistics, including that teens who spend five hours a day or more on devices are 71 per cent more likely to have one risk factor for suicide.[13]

Does Rowan ever spend five hours a day on social media? Do I?

At the start of the pandemic, like many people, I had good intentions about how I would parent. We had the thing, until I went back to nursing at least, that we'd never had before: the gift of time. I retrieved Russian novels from high-up book-shelves and planned to finally work my way through *War and Peace*. I invented 'enrichment hour', and after home-schooling, forced the kids to sit at the table with me for one hour every day while I taught them things that school should but did not teach: how to resuscitate, how tax works, basic car maintenance, fire safety. Rowan and Taylor were willing sports for approximately one week, by which time they'd had enough of real school, and had enough enrichment. 'We don't want to learn how to spot a stroke, or the perils of capitalism, and why credit card companies are thieves', said Rowan. 'We just want to hang out in our rooms, like normal teenagers.'

My son, Tay, nodded a fraction, trying not to insult me with a big nod. 'It's been really great', he said.

Tay was never really a serious gamer and did not have social media on his brick phone yet; so he spent his down time from school playing basketball in the garden. But Ro disappeared to her bedroom, sometimes only coming out to eat, or watch the occasional film, or if I made her get fresh air and exercise, for the best part of a year. I dread to imagine how many hours she must have spent scrolling on social media. I failed to protect her from that, and while being connected to friends at that lonely time was essential, and only available through the means of a phone, I have no doubt she was harmed, too. I never wanted her to have a smartphone at all. My intention was to delay that for as long as possible and turn off the Wi-Fi at night. But by the time the pandemic arrived, Ro was up much later than me (and able to turn the Wi-Fi back on).

I wanted to trust that she'd avoid harmful content and had enough tools to not get addicted to her iPhone, but phones are *designed* to be addictive. We discussed the harmful effects of phone use from the moment the phone conversation came up after Rowan's friend was given an iPhone in primary school. But by the time she was a teenager, she understandably wanted to be in her room or with her friends, either virtually or online. I suspect the pandemic caused phone use to rocket, and, therefore, harm to rocket as well. If the research tells us that over five hours of social media time increases suicidal ideation by such a margin, what is it then for an entire generation of young adults – girls particularly, who consistently fare badly in the research around mental illness and smartphone use – who feasibly spent most of a year or two during the lockdowns scrolling online?

I did not let Rowan have a smartphone until much later than her peers. 'Every single person I know has a mobile phone', she told me from secondary school age onwards. 'Except me.' But even then, I wish I had limited phone time, properly restricted Wi-Fi, insisted, somehow, on time away from technology. I should have tried harder. Knowing what I know now, I am not sure I would have ever let Rowan have a smartphone until adulthood.

Yet. Back then, during the pandemic, when Rowan was fifteen years old, I had returned *War and Peace* to the high bookshelf, and on my days off from the hospital was unable to motivate myself to do anything except watch reality TV. And scroll.

CONVERSATIONS

MOB WIFE ERA

Christie: I'm heading out. Wait – what are you doing? Are you taking a photo of me?

Rowan: Maybe. It's for my album.

Christie: What album?

Rowan: I don't mean to be offensive, but ... you are serving Mob Wife.

Christie: Every sentence you start like that ends up being offensive.

Rowan: *Laughs.* It's for my album. Finally, you're on point. I collect photos of you and your outfits. Me and my friends love them.

Christie: Is there something wrong with my outfits?

Rowan: You're just a bit extra. I mean, you're always wearing that T-shirt that says 'Virginia Woolf'. Or 'Nora Ephron'. You always wear a slogan.

Christie: Isn't that a good thing?

Rowan: You're wearing a leopard-print jumper over a neon vest, and shiny trousers. Purple lipstick.

Christie: Leopard goes with everything.

Rowan: I could jump through those hoop earrings. Are you putting the puppy in your bag?

Christie: She likes it.

Rowan: You do you, hun. Wait – are you going to a work meeting dressed like that?

CHAPTER SIX

I Don't Date Black Girls

Race

Christie: Shall we get a Starbucks?

Rowan: Sure. Or I could make us coffees? I have the syrups.

Christie: I want a Pumpkin Spice.

Rowan: Casper-the-ghost-level white.

Christie: True enough. Did you ever read that original article about pumpkins and white girl privilege, *The Perilous Whiteness of Pumpkins*? It's actually pretty interesting, as was the backlash, then the backlash to the backlash . . .

Rowan: Cool. We should nickname you Pumpkin Spice, you love it so much.

Christie: I think that nickname is problematic.

Rowan: My older sister calls me Birth Control.

Christie: Fair point. Anyway, I'm going to Starbucks; are you coming with me?

Rowan: No thanks. But I'll take a Caramel Frappuccino, extra cream. Thanks, Kraken.

Christie: I rather you call me Pumpkin Spice than Kraken.

Rowan: Cool.

Christie

My former colleague and friend has a son the same age as my son Tay. We live in the same area and our sons attend the same school. They like each other and used to be close friends, but they've drifted apart. Still mates. But they don't go to parties together or hang around with the same group. They no longer hang out much at all. It happened slowly, friendship groups separating like driftwood, and of course it happens to all teens as their identity changes and reforms, creeping towards their adult selves.

My friend and I are super close as ever and love where we live in South London for many reasons. Our sons' school is wonderful. We often talk about how great it is for inclusivity and diversity. It's in one of the best parts of London, with none of the segregation I've experienced in other cities. But although you can walk down my street and see every single type of person and hear a multitude of languages and dialects, as my children go through life, I am starting to see wide cracks.

It occurred to me recently that my son's current friendship group is entirely made up of Black kids. My friend's son's group is – now that my son has jumped ship – entirely white.

'Why don't you go out with them at the weekend? There's a party, I think.'

'There's always a party.' He laughs. 'Every week. Then they'll hang out in the park, drinking and smoking weed in the middle of the night.'

'I mean, it can't be easy being nearly sixteen and not bowing to peer pressure. Going your own way. I'm actually very glad you don't drink and smoke. But it doesn't mean you can't be friends with other kids who do teenage things. Just do your own thing. They're a nice bunch, the group you used to hang around with. Lovely kids. They won't think less of you for not drinking if they are.'

'I know that.' He is quiet for a few moments, trying to articulate something neither of us fully understands. 'But in a park in the middle of the night scenario, they only have to worry about not getting too drunk. Or getting caught smoking weed. We have different things to worry about. If the group does get caught with weed, it's me who gets arrested. And if there's any problems with other kids – it's me who gets stabbed.'

I am ashamed of my ignorance. Before having children who are mixed race or dual heritage – or Black in their eyes and in the eyes of the world – I had never really understood what a racist society we live in. I'd never examined my own bias or thought much about the times in my life when I'd been unintentionally racist. The truth is that I didn't see it, often because it didn't directly affect me. An uncomfortable fact. I see it now. Everywhere. The intersection of race and gender plays out in society daily, and white women, as a rule, have enormous power and wealth. I benefit from living in a structure that makes simply living dangerous for my children. It is high time that white people (like me) 'shine our eyes'.

I go to a friend's wedding – in a diverse area of London – that is entirely white. I go to another friend's party in New York; she is wealthy and everyone at the party is white, but all the staff serving champagne and canapés are Black. I start to notice two tiers everywhere I look. I write this today from the British Library, where the security guards are exclusively Black. I begin to Google company boards and see the faces of trustees – regardless of how diverse a company or organisation seems – a sea of white. Every book event I ever do is like a rally. It is rare to see people of colour in the audience of literary festivals, yet the writers they come to see are from every background. I can't get my head around this.

Segregation is alive and well, and exists in all areas of the UK, even central London, where things are apparently diverse.

Nobody has ever called me terrible names or told me I'm brown and dirty and disgusting at the swing park. Nobody has told me to 'go back to where you came from' or fetishised my body or excluded me from whole class parties or followed my mum to nursery school while I was four years old and laid out British National Party (BNP) leaflets the entire route, like sinister breadcrumbs. Nobody has told me, 'Black people are disgusting thieves', or followed me around and accused me of stealing, or laughed at my name, or consistently touched my hair, called it 'fuzzy' or 'wiry' or 'bushy'. No group of grown men have racially attacked me when I was a young child, or surrounded me when I was a teenager, shouting monkey noises, threatening to kill me.

Nobody has spat on me at a bus stop.

But these things have happened to my children.

I hardly used to think about race, but I now think about it deeply. All white people should. All families like mine must. Our world is full of inequality; our family set-up is not unique. The *Guardian* reports that the 2021 census revealed a 25 per cent increase of households with members of more than one ethnicity.[14] Refinery29 revealed that people with mixed ethnicity now make up the fastest growing population in the UK.[15] (. The 2021 census also showed that 85.9 per cent of lone parents are women. In single-parent families, like ours, where there is a white mum and dual heritage or Black children, conversations about race always come from different life experiences. Research from the Evidence for Equality National Survey in Racism and Ethnic Inequality in a Time of Crisis found that one in six ethnic minority people have experienced a racist physical assault and a third have experienced racial discrimination on education and employment.[16] How do I prepare my children for the realities of a world that my white privilege places me outside of?

Thinking about their Blackness is not enough. It's an examination of my own whiteness that is my work. I belong to a system of privilege that is only afforded to white people. At times, it's uncomfortable thinking about my whiteness as a concept, and the idea that accomplishments and achievements are often more about race than talent and merit. That I am a professor, for example, when the *Independent* reported that in 2020/2021 just 1 per cent of UK professors were Black.[17]. As a white woman, my experience of the world is not the experience of others and not the same experience as my daughter's. Structural racism has benefitted all white people – including me. My children live in a different reality to mine. There is no doubt at all that racism has contributed to Rowan's mental health struggles. How could it not? Luckily, with Black friends, open conversations, and an inclusive network, Ro is starting to unpack, and so am I. We talk often about race, and when it feels uncomfortable, I try and lean into that, and know something is working.

Recovering from mental health issues is not linear. Perhaps, it is not actually possible at all, and like a chronic disease, it will be something that Rowan learns to live with rather than fully recovers from. We all have periods of feeling healthier or not, both physically and mentally, and Rowan seemed to be in a calm phase. She was chatty, and cracking jokes sometimes, and on those days my heart could burst with hope, whatever the conversation.

'I saw this clip from a programme the other day that said nothing is more dangerous than a liberal white woman', Rowan said. She was eating a croissant from a brown paper bag to avoid getting crumbs on the sofa.

We were watching a documentary about Trump. 'Surely he is', I pointed out.

'He's a product of white supremacy, sure. But at least it's obvious. And you're not dangerous unless you've not had your morning coffee, then maybe. But there are tons of white women in total denial about complicity. The world is full of Beckys, or even worse, Karens.'

I've heard the term 'Karen' and understood it to be a derogatory term to mean a woman complaining to managers. 'Surely "Karen" is a sexist term. I actually feel sorry for my cousin, who is called Karen . . .'

Rowan nodded. 'Not the best. We had this discussion in my first secondary school about racism and at least four white girls started crying.'

It is true that when I spoke to my white women friends about race, many got defensive, or upset. Sometimes angry. I had started asking friends to stop using the term 'colour blind', and an old school friend became very fragile after I had to ask her to not touch my son's hair. She seemed unable to acknowledge it was a microaggression, even after discussion. 'Are you saying I'm being *racist*?' she asked, horrified. Then she turned to my son. 'You don't mind, do you? I love your hair.' I have other white women friends who see nothing at all wrong with wearing an afro wig to a fancy-dress party. It really pisses me off, and I actively call out racism when I see it, discuss my concerns, recommend reading and podcasts that I've learnt from, and sometimes, if it persists, walk away from friendships. But I have to ask myself if I would have been them had I not witnessed some of the experiences my children. I hope not.

'What's the answer?' I asked Ro. 'Can you please get a plate?'

'The answer is for you to work out. It is not my job to tell you.'

Rowan

'I don't like Black girls.'

I was at Sophie's house, and we were sitting with three boys from the school around the corner. Friends of friends. We were fourteen.

'I don't like Black girls', Owen repeated.

I looked around Sophie's living room. It was stuffed full of ornaments that her mum collected. I stared at the crystal animals on a shelf. My eyes were glass.

Sophie and Ellie were not listening. Ellie was busy batting her eyelashes so fast at the boy she was sitting next to that her eyes looked like butterflies. Sophie was snogging her boy: I could see tongues from across the room.

'I don't like Black girls', he said again. To make sure I heard him.

I didn't respond for a while. I mean, how do you respond to that? But, eventually, I said 'OK.'

'Not in a racist way, I'm just not attracted to them, just preference you know?'

'OK.'

'I have no problem with Black people, honestly; I just can't see them that way.'

'OK.'

'I have Black friends and all, I just wouldn't date one.'

I started to laugh, but my laugh sounded like a tin can being kicked down a road. I tried to think of something clever to say. I wanted to tell this boy that he is an all-round average boy, and dull, and he was not tall enough for me. That I didn't need to hear about how he could never date a Black person. I wanted to explain my feelings: that there's nothing wrong with having a preference or type of person that you fancy but excluding an entire race of people you would date is racist.

Growing up as, more often than not, the only Black kid in a room has meant that I've become too comfortable with coddling white people's feelings whenever something is said that clearly holds bias and is followed by the iconic ramble of 'oh I just meant that' or the 'not in a racist way'. Here's a tip: If you must justify what you said in a panicked way, you shouldn't have said it; it was racist – acknowledge that, then move on. Like most things in life, racism is a spectrum and every single one of us will have a bias. But for those of us that prefer not to be bigots, it's subconscious.

I didn't say any of that to the boy, Owen. Instead, I said, 'That's fine. Honestly, I get it, I don't date people who look inbred.'

Racism can still be paralysing. These days, depending on my mood, sometimes I will speak up, or leave, or tell someone to simply piss off. But I'm still not always confident enough to deal with it, especially if it's insidious, under the surface, which it often is. Having Black friends helps. A friendship group of people who really get it. But I'd love to go back and hug my younger self.

I've never really considered myself religious, but when I was younger, my mum gave me this book of prayers and I started praying before bed each night. The book had different prayers on each page, illustrated with colourful pictures of happy scenes. I loved it. I would kneel at the side of my bed and clasp my hands together, read a prayer from the book, then move onto my own. I prayed every single night for the same thing. To be white.

I realise now how fucked up that is. I doubt I was the only Black kid who felt that way growing up in a culture that exclusively celebrated whiteness. I prayed for straight, flicky hair. I prayed to be a Disney Princess (Jasmine was the only brown

Disney Princess then, and even she had perfectly straight hair). Or at least, more similar to anyone I saw on TV or in films or in magazines. This was not long ago. At the time of writing, I am now eighteen. I feel so sad for that little girl. I even feel sorry for that boy Owen. I imagine his life now and in the future. I doubt it's that great. Our entire culture is changing. None of us want to be in rooms populated entirely by older white men, except older white men. There's a long way to go, but I'm hopeful. Black friends have helped me and my identity so much. I have an older sister, Alex, who is Black and proud and there's my Black older cousin, Dele, who is an equally positive role model. Of course, even us three women who the world considers Black experience life differently. I am mixed-race, with a Black dad, and white mum, and am light-skinned, which can be a privilege. Colourism – the disadvantages and discrimination Alex and Dele must deal with on a daily basis – is rife across communities.

Being mixed-race feels to me like an in-between identity, and I don't feel in between anything. I am a light-skinned Black person and do not feel I am denying half of myself to say that, but I guess it's strange that I identify with Blackness not whiteness, despite my white mum raising me. Growing up with a white mum is hard to analyse as I've never known anything else. We have sticky, messy conversations about racial politics, and sometimes I can see she is trying to work out the puzzle of it all: How we fit together, and how she fits into the bigger picture. When I was little, I remember her trying to explain how I was Black and she was white. She took a black coffee, a glass of milk and a spare cup, then poured the white and black liquids into the cup together to show how I had Blackness and whiteness inside me: her and my dad both. Even then, I remember thinking that the mixed-together cup looked nothing at all like the white milk, just a different shade of Black. I'm glad she tried. She moved me to a more diverse school and moved our home so we could live in a more diverse area. She sensed the power of that, even if she couldn't fully grasp why it was so important. I remember some friends telling her she was crazy to be moving towards the city rather than out into leafy suburbs, where money would have gone a lot further. 'Knife crime, gangs, drugs', they would cite. Those things do happen. But despite these inner-city challenges, I think Mum made the right call. Nobody in South London asks me to repeat my surname and asks how it's pronounced time and time and time again. Nobody has ever asked me 'where I'm *really* from'. But this happens everywhere else.

When I look in the mirror these days, I see who I am, and who I am becoming. When people ask me where I'm really from I tell them. I am from South London and Nigeria. I'm from an allotment in Stevenage and a snail farm in Lagos, from jollof rice and Welsh rarebit, and from dance and books and the smell of the seaweed in The Isle of Man. I'm from creativity and neuro-spice and Dumpling Mum. I'm from a pandemic, and sepsis, and Stick n Poke. I'm from five dotted-around siblings, one Black sister, one Muslim brother, another little sister up North, a new stepbrother at Bible College, another who wears a Rolex. I'm from always swimming in freezing cold water, and dancing at the Brit Awards and the snow. I'm from nearly dying a few times, but then surviving after all.

And then I ask them, where are you from?

Things are changing. The world is moving fast and some people are being left behind. But I am ready.

CONVERSATIONS

THE GREATEST GENERATION
July 1953

Maternal Great-Grandmother: I've run you a bath, love. It's so good to have you back home. I missed you so. Two long years! *Cries, quietly.*

Maternal Great-Grandfather: There, there woman, I'm back now. Come on, don't cry. *Hugs her then disappears into bathroom.*

Maternal Great-Grandmother: Here's a fresh towel, love. What's that?

Maternal Great-Grandfather: What?

Maternal Great-Grandmother: On your chest. Above your heart. What is that?

Maternal Great-Grandfather: Ah, it's nothing.

Maternal Great-Grandmother: It looks like a scar. A big one. What happened? Tom? you're scaring me.

Maternal Great-Grandfather: Come on, love, there's nothing to worry about. *Hugs her again.* I'm here now. It's just a scratch. That's all. *Whispers.* From when I got shot in Korea.

Maternal Great-Grandmother: *Gasps.* You got shot? You got shot in the chest and you didn't tell me?

Maternal Great-Grandfather: I didn't want to worry you, love. I'm fine. Strong as an ox.

Maternal Great-Grandmother: *Crying.* What happened?

Maternal Great-Grandfather: You know when I sent a telegram to say I was in Korea and unable to write? Well, I was in the military hospital. In Japan. There a few months.

Maternal Great-Grandmother: You could have died. You didn't tell me. Shot! In the heart!

Maternal Great-Grandfather: Only you could shoot me in the heart, Mary. This was just a scratch.

Maternal Great-Grandmother: You should have told me. I'm your wife.

Maternal Great-Grandfather: I didn't want you to worry, love. It's nothing.

WAR

Rowan: If NATO goes to war with Russia, we're going to be conscripted, apparently.

Christie: Hi Ro. Your number didn't come up on my phone. Where are you?

Rowan: With a friend. Doesn't matter. Did you hear me? We're going to actual war?

Christie: I think it's highly unlikely that you will be called up to the front line any time soon. Are you back for dinner? I'm making a veggie curry and tarka daal.

Rowan: This is serious. But yes to tarka daal. Doubt we'll get that on the front line.

Christie: Ro, you can't think that any government in the world would send you and your friends to war. I mean, think about that.

Rowan: I thought it sounded a bit strange. All war is horrific, but this has blown up on TikTok. So many people are sending memes and reasons Gen Z can't go to war. Hang on, I'll read some:

How will I get Greg's pizza slices in trenches?
I have sensory issues. The sound of gunfire is a no-no.
I literally cannot live without acrylic nails.
I take Fridays as mental health days every week, so I'll go but Fridays are duvet days.
I do not suit camouflage. Ick.

If Deliveroo and Uber are not available to me, my performance will be poor.

I have a skincare routine that requires a mini-fridge.

Christie: *Laughing a bit.* I like that you're able to laugh at yourselves. Honestly, there is no way Gen Z will be going to war. In seriousness, it would surely never align with your values.

Rowan: Exactly that. Patriotism is dead. Nobody my age will support a government like ours or kill innocent people for political nonsense. Also, I'm an asthmatic vaper, so probably couldn't go anyway on medical grounds.

Christie: Stop vaping. Please. And you do not have asthma.

Rowan: The war office doesn't know that. I can wheeze on demand. Got to go, they're doing one-pound-a-shot happy hour.

Christie: Bye, Ro. *Whispers.* God help us all.

CHAPTER SEVEN

Future Dread

Existential Threats

Christie: Hi Mr Dimitri, it's Rowan's Mum again. Can you talk?

Mr Dimitri: Of course. I hope things are OK? We haven't seen Rowan today yet, I'm afraid . . . How is she? And how are you?

Christie: Well, it's eventful. Do you know about the tattooing?

Mr Dimitri: What do you mean tattooing?

Christie: Stick n Poke.

Mr Dimitri: I'm not following. Is Rowan OK?

Christie: She's safe. She's in her bedroom. I'll do my best to get her to lessons somehow this afternoon, but at the moment she's refusing to move and says she's having a really bad mental health episode.

Mr Dimitri: I'm sorry to hear that. Can we do anything? Do you want me to talk with her?

Christie: I don't think she would. But I do need to let you know about the tattoos. The latest craze. Sick n Poke . . .

Mr Dimitri: She hasn't got a tattoo, has she?

Christie: They all have. The whole friendship group.

Mr Dimitri: *Silence.*

Christie: Apparently, they've been tattooing themselves, and each other. I'm not sure if other parents have mentioned anything.

Mr Dimiti: Nothing. Tell me they're temporary. Henna?

Christie: Nope.

Mr Dimitri: *Silence.*

Christie: Rowan is covered. They got tattoo kits online. I mean, the infection risk is what worries me most despite how bad they look.

Mr Dimitri: This is a new one. *Sighs.*

Christie: Indeed.

Mr Dimitri. What did you call it, stick?

Christie: Stick n Poke. It's an internet craze, apparently.

Mr Dimitri: *Sad voice.* Oh my.

Christie: I know.

Mr Dimitri: Thanks for letting us know. Please send my best to Rowan. I am around all afternoon if she makes it in.

Christie: Thank you.

Mr Dimitri: Honestly, I'm sorry. I really hope you are OK. I'll investigate this. Take care of yourself. What a stressful time for you and Rowan.

Christie

Rowan was always writing on things she shouldn't have. Back when she could first hold a pen, she'd mark her territory. She was four or five when she wrote 'Bella' on every item of furniture in her room, with a Sharpie. When questioned about it, she denied all knowledge and blamed her brother, who was a toddler and barely able to hold his head up, let alone a pen. 'He wrote my name on everything', she said, 'so you would think it was me.' I banned pens in the house, but she'd always find one. Another day she came downstairs with two giant thick black eyebrows drawn in perfect arches over her own. It didn't wash off and she looked shocked for a few months. I always assumed she'd grow out of it and not for one minute that she'd write on her own skin, permanently.

She'd been wearing long sleeves for a few days and it was hot. I wondered if she'd self-harmed, which I worried about all the time. But eventually, I bumped into her coming out of the bathroom in a towel and was shocked to discover the word 'Photosynthesize' in uneven letters tattooed across her forearm. On the other arm, a badly drawn teddy bear with wings. It transpired that Rowan was covered in tattoos: her arms, legs, torso, stomach, chest. You can see shock in the air. It changes the shape of nothing, becomes wavy, like a hot day in a desert. I watched the air change shape as I listened. She told me they were all doing it at school, sometimes on themselves, sometimes on each other. 'Temporary', I said. 'Tell me, dear God, they're temporary.'

She went on to show me the 'sterile' needles. A pack full of dust shoved in her sock drawer, containing a dozen or so needles and some black ink in a small squat pot. 'We got it online', she said. 'It's permanent.'

I looked at her, my beautiful, perfect daughter, and tried to figure out why she'd want to do such a thing.

'I don't want to be beautiful', she said. 'At least not by your standards.'

My eyes were so full of tears the tattoos on her arms looked even more blurry. 'You might one day. You will change your mind. That's the point of being sixteen. You get to change your mind about everything.'

'I don't care', she said. Her tone of voice was flat, it was true. She didn't care.

But I worry she will one day. She'll care a lot. Sometimes, parenting Ro is like watching her drowning, throwing her a life jacket, and standing paralysed as she swims in the opposite direction. Sometimes, it is just about hanging on. That's it. There is no magic to raising a teenager other than sheer grit to love them no matter what. My mum must have felt exactly the same parenting me.

I thought a lot about what might have driven Ro to do Stick n Poke. I'm sure some of it was the trend aspect, as it was all over TikTok. But it was more than skin deep. More profound than self-harm. It was not self-hatred or even hatred of the world that propelled her, I suspect, but apathy. She was maybe so overwhelmingly anxious about the state of humanity that she literally didn't see the point in *not* doing it. Permanent didn't exist. Nothing was permanent, not even the planet. The American Psychological Association describes eco-anxiety as a chronic fear of environmental doom.[18] But for Ro, this moment in history was acute not chronic. I'm sure she was worried about climate change, AI, democracy, war, future pandemics. It was hard to reassure her, because her worries were not unfounded. I wondered if I'd have struggled so much with my mental health that I'd have tattooed myself, if I'd been around during Stick n Poke. Probably.

I was, according to my dad, 'banging on about social justice before it was popular'. I'm glad that activism is becoming more commonplace with Generation Z. It wasn't always aspirational, at least not in the shouty way I approached it. I was the only person in my failing secondary school to pick Environmental Science as a GCSE option, but they ran it anyway. I was fascinated by the ozone layer. Fridges and my brother's Lynx Africa solvents disturbed me in equal measures, and I spent many hours discussing such matters with my science teacher one-on-one, who tried desperately to integrate me into the 'normal' science class. I was undeterred. I pinned my Campaign for Nuclear Disarmament badge to my chest and marched into heated debates about fossil fuels and the plight of polar bears. I wanted to discuss likely environmental catastrophes and, at that time, it made me deeply unpopular with my peers, who wanted to talk instead about who got off with who and what arguments had broken out in the friendship group. I was consumed by thoughts of activism. But I found my people in any case. I dated an unemployed man named Ulysses, who lived in a shed, smoked an incredible amount of hash, and talked non-stop about the Amazon Rainforest. I paired up with a friend and we travelled to a few working men's clubs in Scotland, for reasons unclear to me now. My friend played saxophone while I shouted poetry I'd written about melting ice caps and famine in Ethiopia at men who probably just wanted to drink their beer in peace. I once threw a pot of paint in Stevenage town centre on a woman who was wearing a fur coat. 'It's fake', she shouted, chasing me down the road. 'How dare you, you little shit. I love animals.'

It's so interesting to me, reflecting on the person I was then, and thinking about who I am now. Of course I recycle and try and avoid plastic where I can. I am increasingly conscious of carbon offsetting. On the whole, I buy local, in-season food and avoid fast fashion. All the usual 'doing my bit' things. But if I'd been born when Rowan was, I'd have no doubt been chaining myself to fracking railings or lying on a proposed new airport runway. I would have self-harmed, I'm certain, and I also would have got on board with Stick n Poke. When Rowan does something I totally disapprove of, I often remind myself that I would likely have done the same.

Would it have simply been more performative? I liked to shout but aside from chucking paint on some poor animal lover, I was not an activist of much action. I'm even quieter about things now, and if I want to attempt to change people's minds or hearts, to call people to arms, or simply highlight something sitting in darkness, I use my pen. It feels far more effective.

But I fear in losing some of the anger of youth, I've lost the energy to care quite as deeply about important things. As I get older, sometimes wiser, occasionally humbler, life is far less intense, and I like that stability. But with intensity comes passion, for people and for causes. At times I feel less connected to the universe. It's not apathy, though plenty of times I have been familiar with the most dangerous of emotions, that is, no emotion at all. When facing existential threats of every nature, it's hard not to be overwhelmed to the point of numbness: climate change, pandemics, war, and, increasingly, AI.

'It's us and us, not us and them', I told Rowan, at every opportunity.

'Not for long', she muttered.

We were sitting at the orthodontist, which was a frequent event for us. Like so many teens, Rowan's teeth were growing in unruly directions, and one tooth stuck so high up, her dentist described it as *fused into her skull*. 'We might need to just leave it there', he said, which had Ro fake-gagging a little.

The waiting room was full of teenagers slumped over their phones and parents next to them, mothers mostly, also slumped over their phones. Nobody spoke or even looked at each other. Every now and then, a dental nurse came in and shouted a name and a different pair sloped into the large treatment room.

'What do you mean not for long?'

'Your argument that there is only us and us. You're talking about humans.'

I peered at Ro's phone as she talked. She was in a phase of watching textures. Jelly, sponge, slime. I flashed back to her as a toddler, her hands in buckets of soapy water, or sand, or making mud pies in the garden.

She scrolled. 'AI will be the end of that', she said. 'There'll be an us and them.' She looked up briefly, then back to her phone. 'There already is.'

I wondered if she was right. Certainly, Rowan spoke a language that I was partially outside of. As a Generation X woman, or Xennial, that is someone born on the cusp of millennial and Gen X, I have partially grown up in a culture of technology. But I can also remember the before. Gen Z is the first generation for whom there is no before and after in that sense, just after and after from now on. That creates a dividing line between generations that we have not seen before. A language barrier. There is also perhaps something more worrying about the threats future generations are experiencing, because they are perhaps unseen, in our society at least. My grandparents literally went to war. My grandad was shot. And yet, to my knowledge, he never experienced the overwhelming dread and anxiety that Ro's generation experiences about the future of the planet. Fear is surely always worse when the enemy is unknown.

'It might be AI that causes the end of the world', Ro told me as she held her phone out in front of her, showing a photograph of the earth taken from space. 'Or climate change. These brown patches are basically pollution. The planet is dying.'

For a long time, the media has been reporting climate change as code red for humanity. Every week we are bombarded with more catastrophic news. In February 2024 alone the UN reported that exploitation has left species crucial to the survival of our planet on the edge of extinction. The BBC announced that polar bears, as my anxiety predicted thirty years ago, are dying of starvation as ice melts.[19] The world has breached the crucial 1.5 degrees Celsius warming threshold for a full year, the first time in history.[20] Of course, nothing happens in isolation, and the dance between war and climate has never been fiercer. The International Committee of the Red Cross reports that climate change worsens vulnerabilities, deepens inequalities, and can exacerbate factors that contribute to tensions. Meanwhile, the *Guardian* reports that nearly 15 per cent of Americans don't believe climate change is real.[21]

'What's the point of school?' Rowan asked. 'What's the point of anything? The world is literally on fire, and you want me to go to my tap-dancing class?'

When Greta Thunberg decided Fridays were for school strikes, Ro was way ahead of her already. Her attendance by that point was 21 per cent. The *Telegraph* reported that in 2023, 140,000 children were classed as 'severely absent' from school – meaning they missed at least 50 per cent of their lessons – an increase of 134 per cent since the pandemic.[22]

Rowan sailed so close to being expelled. I would be at school all the time having meetings with educational psychologists, teachers, pastoral care teams. Rowan, meanwhile, spent entire days in bed, sometimes, underneath the weight of it all. It felt like forever while we were going through it. But all of life is seasonal. Eventually, after taking to her bed for months, in the manner of a wealthy Victorian Lady, she got up.

It came from her, not me, her recovery. Even therapy and help from CAMHS, and support from school and community made little difference in Rowan's case to her mental health. It was internal, her struggle, and so was recovery.

There were some small things I did do though that I feel

helped me, and helped her. I made a conscious choice to show up for her exactly as I am. I wanted Rowan to know me intimately. All of me. The good bits and the terrible bits, in order that she feel safe enough to show me exactly who she is. I want to know Rowan. All of her. To encourage her to show up fully, as herself. That makes for a fiery relationship at times. But a completely honest one.

During the bleakest of times, when Ro's future looked grim, I kept reminding her, and myself, that day always follows night. The Sun always shines after rain. *This too will pass*. Even this.

I am so grateful for Ro. To know exactly who she is feels like the greatest of gifts.

Rowan

Humanity's response to existential threats is an absolute disaster. We've known about climate change and its impending catastrophe for decades, yet what have we done? Squabbled over trivialities, ignored scientists' warnings, and let greed and politics dictate our actions. It's infuriating to see leaders bicker and dawdle while our planet burns. And don't even get me started on the so-called climate deniers who refuse to face reality or the corporations profiting from the destruction of our environment.

It's like watching a slow-motion train wreck, except we're all passengers and nobody seems to care enough to pull the emergency brake.

The prospect of AI as a threat to humanity is another chilling reality. Without robust safeguards and ethical guidelines, we risk creating a future where AI becomes a force that threatens our very existence.

The words above were written by ChatGPT, not me.

I had more than one friend at school who wrote every single piece of coursework using ChatGPT. I think about that a lot. It changes everything, in terms of learning, education, purpose. If my friends can do that already, what will the landscape of school, and university, look like for the next generation? What was the point? What's the point of anything? But of course, AI is not my only, or even necessarily biggest, concern. It's a time of existential threat pick n mix.

Climate dread is growing amid Gen Z especially. Our world is quite literally on fire, and yet the conversations we have with older people about what we want to be when we grow up are almost laughable. Alive. That's what young people aspire to be.

Living in a world where catastrophic fires and storms and tsu-
namis are not causing the biggest refugee crisis in our living
history. We would rather not be extinct, thanks. I read a 2021
study on young people's voices on climate anxiety by Caroline
Hickman and others, who found that more than 50 per cent of
16- to 25-year-olds feel humanity is doomed.[23]

Meanwhile, I was meant to attend my tap-dancing class?

Instead, like many teenagers now, I stopped eating, sleeping,
and going to lessons. Instead, my friends and I smoked a lot of
weed in the woods next to school and began tattooing each
other. One day, after three days of feeling manic and no sleep at
all, I tattooed the word 'Photosynthesize' onto my forearm in
the changing room at school. I have no idea why I chose that
word; I don't remember thinking about plants and nature, more
how I didn't care what was written on my skin, and |I didn't
care if I lived or died, that in the end, we'd all return to the
earth. There was something else, too. I felt everything was so
out of control – my head, the world, the future – that I wanted
to claim my own body. I was in control of my body. I could do
with my own skin whatever I wanted.

Mum went ballistic, of course, but when she calmed down,
she was so sad. She said Stick n Poke, and especially the way
I did it, was a form of self-harm. I didn't see it like that, more
a form of not caring. But the relief in expressing myself in
that way was short-lived. I felt worse, not better. It was after
the tattooing phase that I stopped going to school. Some days
my mental health was so bad I literally couldn't brush my
teeth. I didn't have the mental energy to do anything but cry,
sleep, cry some more. I felt totally and utterly empty of
motivation.

'Please, Rowan, please.' Mum was hovering in my bedroom
doorway wearing her dressing gown. She had taken to getting
up at seven to begin the process of coming into my room and
gently cajoling me to get up.

Half an hour later, she'd return. Sometimes with coffee. She'd try to sit on the edge of the bed and talk softly to me. 'It's really important you get up for school. It's Wednesday already and you haven't been in at all.'

'What's the point?' I said. 'What is the actual fucking point?'

Another half an hour. 'Rowan, I'll drive you, and I'll collect you, if it helps?'

I ignored her. I wanted to close my eyes and check out. No wonder so many people I knew were taking ketamine. I wanted to tranquilise myself, sleep through it.

By noon, the softly gently approach had turned into screaming. 'Get up', she shouted, before aggressively opening the curtains. 'I mean it, Ro. You can't just stay in bed. You will lose your school place. Do you know how lucky you are? How many kids would give their right arm to get a place at The BRIT School? It is a huge privilege to go to a free arts school, and you are wasting your place, wasting a massive opportunity. Get up.'

'I don't care', I shouted back. 'Maybe I'll just stay in bed forever.' I felt my breathing get quicker and quicker. I was never far from a panic attack. I curled up into a ball.

'You seem so overwhelmed', she said, trying visibly to soften herself. 'And terrified. What's going on in your mind? How can I help?'

'I don't want to talk about it', I replied. I didn't have the words. It was hard to articulate that paralysis I felt. I spent my whole time and energy trying not to think about killing myself, if I could think that day at all. Every time someone would subtly remind me of apparently all I had to live for, a list would appear in my head: war, or climate, or AI, and slavery, colonialism, past and present genocide. The Big Things. And that was without the idea of joblessness, cost of living, and the prospect of never being able to own my own house in my lifetime. I tried to focus on my breathing, or distract myself with

TikTok, or *Grey's Anatomy*. But suicidal thoughts swirled around my head, until my brain was a washing machine full of dread.

'Ro', Mum whispered. Then louder, 'Ro, you need to go to school.'

I sat up a bit and stared at her. She looked awful. Her eyes were red from crying and worry. I wanted to say I was sorry, and hug her, but even though she was sitting right there on my bed, she felt so far away. It was like living behind glass that might break and shatter at any moment. 'There are some things', I told her, 'that are more important than school.'

Mum got up and slammed the door behind her, and I heard her phone the school to say she didn't know what to do and I wouldn't be in. 'The only reason I can give is that she's mentally unwell', she said.

I felt hopeless. Overwhelmed. Becoming an adult was a terrifying prospect, the idea of having to face responsibilities regardless of what was happening in the wider world. It annoyed me that the responsibility of finding the solution to so many problems that older generations have caused rests on young people. The heavy lifting of world issues seems to have been laid on the shoulders of teenagers. I wanted peace amidst all this madness. I needed to go to sleep and wake up when the world was a bit better, and when I no longer wanted to end myself.

The world is no better, but I got better anyway. Many things helped me with healing. My friends. Time. Growing up. And my mum. She didn't help at first, but after I started helping myself, she was essential. She didn't understand, but even then, she just always loved me despite that. Constant love is a powerful force.

Something shifted as time went on. I was sitting on the grass and the sun was out. I remember its warmth on my skin and realising that I felt good. Somehow, all those thoughts that had once crushed me seemed smaller. I started to take in the world once again, the good and the bad.

I turned to anger. It is far easier, it turns out, to work with anger rather than apathy. I used to think that my voice was so small there was no point using it, and most of the time, I was too unwell to engage in future dread about humanity. But I began to follow activists like Mikaela Loach and Greta Thunberg and think about movements like 4B, which originated in South Korea after the #MeToo movement and rejected sex and marriage with men. I found a community on social media that was not, this time, exploring darkness but searching for light. I began to remember the feeling of sun on my skin. Instead of hiding in my bed, one day, I felt well enough to stand up.

Mum was downstairs the first day I got out of bed and managed to shower. She was working at the kitchen table, a steaming coffee next to her. She looked up in surprise to see me out of bed before noon. 'Hi! You look a bit brighter.'

I put the kettle on then sat down next to her. 'I have therapy at 1', I said.

'How do you feel about that?' Mum was desperately trying not to pry, but her name may well have been Pry Pry as well as Cray Cray. She couldn't help it.

'I don't want to talk about that', I said.

She swiftly changed the subject. 'I was listening to the news again just now. There's a bird, type of parrot in Australia near the wildfires, that has started making the sound of sirens. Birds that imitate fire engines. So sad.'

'Well, the world is literally on fire.'

Mum nodded. 'Maybe we could go on an XR march together? This feels like a much better response to life than refusing to go to school or tattooing yourself. Do you think that's what's getting you down? Future dread? Worrying about the state of the world is surely making young people mentally unwell.'

I looked at Mum in horror. Imagined her wearing double leopard print on a march, taking selfies of us and handing out Wagon Wheels. 'I'm not feeling up to crowds. I'm not trying to avoid school, or intending to lie there thinking about climate change or AI. I literally just wanted to die half the time. Also, I always told you I would get tattoos.'

'Hmm. Well, I worry all the time about the big things. Mostly climate change, I guess. Do you remember when I was writing my first novel? You were quite little then, but I had to research all about the politics of oil', Mum said. She had this way of surprising me. For someone who could never remember the Netflix password, she had a lot of information in her head. 'Anyway, I'm glad you're feeling a fraction better today. Checking out of life is never the answer.'

'You're wrong about that. It's not your answer, but it was mine. Checking out of life for a while was not a waste at all. I needed it. I wanted to die.'

Mum blinked back tears.

I hugged her. She squeezed me so hard I could barely breathe. 'I did want to die, but now I don't', I said. 'Can you stop bear-hugging me so tightly?'

She let me go, and we stood and looked at each other, and I noticed her holding back tears. 'This is weird and creepy', I said.

She smiled. 'Totally. Coffee?'

I nodded and got a mug out, shaking instant coffee into it without using a spoon. Exactly like Mum does.

CONVERSATIONS

MOON WATER

Christie: Will you please turn the lights off? You've left the bathroom light on again, and the one in your room.

Rowan: I'm going back up.

Christie: If you didn't have the curtains closed the entire time, you would have this thing called daylight.

Rowan: I am a night creature.

Christie: Ridiculous. Let some light in. You'll get rickets at this rate, you're probably so Vitamin D deficient.

Rowan: I take your supplements. Wait, did you mean to style your hair like that? You look a bit like Margaret Thatcher.

Christie: That's what I was going for.

Rowan: *Shrugs.* Each unto their own, I guess.

Christie: Of course that wasn't what I was going for. Ro. Go up now, turn your light off, and open your curtains. Or I'll do it.

Rowan: You can't. I have Moon Water in there and you will void it if it is exposed to daylight.

Christie: What on earth is Moon Water?

Rowan: You wouldn't understand.

Christie: Try me.

Rowan: You asked why I was in the garden at 4 a.m. Well, that's why. I was collecting Moon Water. It would be good for you, to be honest. As a Virgo, if you collected Moon Water from a Cancer Moon, it would most likely move you from intellectualisation to emotion.

Christie: I don't understand.

Rowan: Exactly.

Christie: *Sighs.* Turn the light off.

Rowan: I'm a vampire. This is how we live. Byeeee. Wait, did you buy any avocados?

CHAPTER EIGHT

Ancient Greek Civilisation

Class

Rowan: I'm going to university to study classical history.

Christie: What do you mean, Classics? Where did that come from? You've been dancing your whole life . . .

Rowan: I've always been fascinated with ancient Greek civilisation.

Christie: Since when?

Rowan: I've got lots of obsessions. I'm obsessive. Like you.

Christie: That's true. It just feels a bit leftfield. How exciting. Wait, do you need to speak Greek or Latin?

Rowan: I'll learn one. Probably Greek.

Christie: I can't believe it. How wonderful!

Rowan: The professor swore in the interview. That's how I knew it was right.

Christie: You're basing your decision about the next few years and possible future career on the fact that a professor accidentally swore during your interview?

Rowan: Yup.

Christie: Jolly good. Incidentally, what career does Classical Studies lead to? Have you thought ahead?

Rowan: Nope. *Pulls out* The Iliad.

Christie: I'm pleased for you, Ro. This is a curveball that we couldn't have even imagined a year ago . . .

Rowan: You can go now. *Glances up. Smiles.*

Christie: I can go now. *Doesn't move.*

Christie

When Rowan turned ten – double digits – I gave her the choice of taking her for a short trip away or a party with her friends. 'Rome', she said, as though she was Audrey Hepburn in *Roman Holiday*. 'I want to go to Rome.'

It occurred to me, as we were flying to Rome, Rowan eating a Pret sandwich and reading a book I'd bought her at the airport, that along with race, we had a significant difference between us. I grew up very working class, and even though as a single mum I often struggled for money during her early years, Rowan was being raised in a middle-class world that I could have never imagined at her age. Class sometimes gave me and Ro different languages, a complex mix of alternative views about aspiration, security, work ethic, and expectation. Of course there was nothing at all romantic about poverty, but when I entered the middle classes, I felt as though I was learning a new set of rules to a game I didn't much like.

Writing gave me friends from all class backgrounds, and I was surprised to find that some upper-class people – aristocratic, old-monied – had much in common with those from my working-class roots. My working-class friends had no money to buy things, and the old-money wealthy people I sometimes met in the writing world had all the money in the world and, therefore, could buy anything they wanted; so there was no real significance at either end of the class spectrum for *stuff*. I noticed other similarities, too, between my working-class and posh friends: old-fashioned manners, straightforward, sometimes blunt, talking, trusting that the feral kids would come home when hungry, bohemian chaos, a couple of small presents for Christmas and birthdays – all that smelled like home. My friends from both these classes were walkers, heavy drinkers, thrifty, proper cooks. Nobody had a Peloton or believed in 'wellness'. When I moved from a very poor area to a more affluent one, just before I became pregnant with Rowan, I discovered that the first question people asked me was what job I did, and the second question was what job my husband did. So many of the middle-class school mums there seemed to be obsessed with the acquisition of things. I didn't feel much affinity to my new crowd. It all felt a bit alien to me.

Despite all my complex feelings, moving away from where I grew up and ending up in the middle classes has afforded me and the children immense privilege. There we were en route to Rome as her birthday present.

Long before she could speak, Rowan could dance. She seemed to have an innate natural ability to move her body to express herself. That, combined with a musical ear, fearlessness, and excellent muscle memory, gifted her an ability that neither me nor her dad possessed. I was thrust into another world. Rowan joined her first dance school, ballet, at age two, and from then until the pandemic hit when she was fourteen, I ferried her around, waiting for hours in the car, spending, no doubt, thousands of pounds on lessons and travel and uniform and costumes. Dance was a circle of middle-class privilege. Like many of my friends' kids, her life was one of clubs and opportunities and activities. Even when she was a baby, before dance, I took her to music class and art class and baby yoga. The babies lay on the floor on mats while the mums danced around them shaking tambourines. I once took Rowan's paternal grandmother, who was over visiting from Nigeria, to the music class. She asked me how much it cost, and then rolled her eyes, stating that it was ridiculous.

'Ridiculous' was a word that I encountered from all the older women in my family. I'm always waiting for it to slip out of my mouth when I talk to Rowan. It will surely come.

'Why are we here so early?'

'To get to the front. Plus, it's free on the first Wednesday of every month, so the hotel warned of a long queue.'

We were outside Vatican City, at the very front, bar three nuns. Rowan was bored already, but I had promised ice cream on the Spanish Steps after this visit. It was hot, and I hadn't thought to bring water. Organisation was never my forte. We waited and waited and waited and eventually they opened the doors.

'Walk fast', I said. 'And don't look back.'

Rowan didn't question me. She knew the plan. The night before, while we were eating what she describes to this day as the best pasta of her life, I had told her that the building and each room were so incredible that people going in would stop in each section to stare at the brilliance of it all. 'But it's the Sistine Chapel I want to take you to. I know how much you'll love it. If we run, or at least walk quickly, we might just be the only ones in there before the crowds.'

We were the first. We had a good ten minutes or so, just me and Rowan, standing in the Sistine Chapel and looking up at the ceiling. You could hear a pin drop. It felt so spiritual, and I was moved to tears.

But when I looked at Rowan, she was hopping from foot to foot and looking at the floor. 'My neck hurts', she said. 'Can we go and have ice cream?'

I laughed. 'Sure thing.' She liked the Sistine Chapel, but she loved the pasta. Like dance, she often loved things that I did not understand. She always went her own way and often surprised me, even then.

Later that trip, we visited the Pantheon. I said we could leave after ten minutes and get some pasta. But Rowan simply stared at it. Her eyes were open wide. 'I don't want to go yet', she said. 'It's miraculous.'

Rowan

Being a dancer is never easy, but being a dancer during a global pandemic was impossible. I tried following lessons, tap-dancing around my bedroom, keeping up with ballet and a toned-down version of contemporary. I'd spent years learning technique, both at The BRIT School, where I danced full time, and as part of the Centre for Advanced Training at Trinity Laban. I always loved dancing. I used to explain things to Mum using my body instead of words. I'd dance out things to her that I found hard to articulate. She would look confused; after all, it was a strange language to her, but I thought in dance as well as words. When I could no longer dance, I thought the world would end. But then I remembered a dream from long ago, a trip to Rome for my tenth birthday, a building that was full of ghosts and stories.

When I recovered from mental illness, I began to read again. I spent a year immersed in stories and myths from the ancient world and read my way through so many greats: Homer, Plato, Aristotle, Virgil. I was hooked. I felt that I'd opened a door to another universe, a world so far away from our contemporary one, yet close enough that the more I read of the past, the more sensory the experience became. Reading the Classics took me from my bedroom and enabled me to time-travel. I'd spent ages trying to get out of my head, but it was only by going into my head that I found peace. The best kind of escapism. I didn't need to leave my body anymore. I could stay right inside it and go back to the beginning. I didn't need to act out tragedies with my friends. I could read them.

Mum was beside herself with excitement and couldn't contain it. She was almost dancing her way through the aisles in IKEA,

chucking in bedsheets and lamps and cushions and cutlery. I
pushed the trolley and watched her.

'You'll need mugs at uni', she said. 'Grey or blue. How many?
Do you want half a dozen?'

A few other teenagers walked past pushing trolleys, their
own mums dancing around them. A rite of passage. 'Six? Why
the hell would I need six mugs?'

'Well, if you have friends 'round for tea. Or coffee. You need
to be able to offer them a drink.'

'Mum, nobody my age drinks tea, and nobody has six friends
over to their room in halls for a cup of tea. I think you are imagining a period drama, not university life.'

She smiled, linked her arm through mine, and we walked on.
'Meatballs?' Every now and then she held up a toilet brush or
mattress protector and I shook my head. But when she lifted a
cosy bedspread, I nodded. She threw it into the trolley,
delighted. 'That will be so cuddly', she said. 'You'll be lovely
and toasty warm.'

We got some veggie meatballs and sat down to eat. She went
back three times for more lingonberry sauce, I noticed, and
always struck up a conversation with whoever was getting
ketchup. She is such an oddbod, my mum, but I realised, all of
a sudden, how much I would miss her.

'You seem so excited about IKEA. Next level.'

She laughed. 'You don't understand', she said, and her laugh
dropped away.

'Try me.'

She looked a bit sad and reached across the table to hold my
hand, which was awkward on a number of levels. But I let her.

'The worst part of the last few years, and there were lots of
worst parts, was seeing all your peers do things. All my friends'
children who you grew up with, the same age. Taking driving
lessons and passing their test. Going to university open days.
Sweet-sixteen birthday parties. Ordinary things. It wasn't

jealousy, it was pain. Seeing you miss out. Normal things. Events that I never saw happening for you. I just saw everyone living their lives, and you not living your life. Like you had pressed stop on it all. Mental illness had. I thought that might be forever. And look where we are. I am so, so proud of you. More than you'll ever know.'

I let go of Mum's hands, after giving them a squeeze, and ate a chip. 'You're so soppy.'

She wiped a tear away with the back of her hand and smiled again. 'Remember when we had a huge argument in front of the psychiatrist.'

I laughed. 'OMG, so funny. Poor guy didn't know what to do.'

After she paid the hefty IKEA bill, due to a trolley full of crap I most likely would not need, we went outside, and I rolled a cigarette. Mum took out her phone and took endless photos of me smoking a roll-up, balancing on a trolley outside IKEA, as if I had just climbed the highest mountain in the world, and we had reached the summit.

Growing up, I didn't really think much about class, but like with all things, I'm a bit of a mash-up. Mum grew up very working class, and my maternal grandparents and all their side of the family were what Mum called 'salt of the earth types'. Meanwhile, my Nigerian grandparents had live-in staff and owned an entire street in Lagos. During my early years, when Mum was working as a nurse and a single parent, we had no money, to the extent that I sellotaped my shoes rather than tell her I had a hole in them because I knew she couldn't afford new school shoes. But later, we moved to a comfortable life of privilege on a leafy road in London. I think it's probably useful to have seen and lived through both sides of the class coin. I do not take money for granted. I am never wasteful. I see the good and bad in both working-class and middle-class systems, and I am aware of a bigger picture of financial inequality.

But Classics can be confronting. At university, I am starting to discover that my perception wasn't that straightforward. Classical Studies is an elitist space. It feels like only certain people are fully prepared to study it – those who've had access to Latin and Greek lessons at school, for example. Not only are Classical Studies for the very few, it seems, but also steeped in problematic history. My professors are almost all white men. I am learning much about the wonderful and rich subject that I've fallen in love with but simultaneously discovering its connection to colonialism, imperialism, and white supremacy. Life gets more confusing the more I understand, which is a bit of a shock. In a way, this duality draws me closer to Classics, instead of pushing me away. I want to wrestle intellectually with complex things. I want to understand nuance. Sometimes, I am so rigid about my ideas that it's hard to change my mind. But I guess that's what adulting is really about: knowing that things can be good and bad at the same time. And so can people.

Connecting to stories, ancient myths and all their characters makes me feel connected to something bigger, more mysterious and miraculous than I can articulate. Less alone.

That's what books can do. That's what I hope this book does for someone else out there. A sixteen-year-old as lost as I was. Or a mum like my mum, whispering *come back to me*. I did come back. I'm here. I exist. I breathe. I hurt and cry and scream and laugh. Instead of feeling nothing, I feel everything. I am really here.

A LETTER TO MY MUM

Mum,

I used to want you to be like other mums. But now I love your randomness. I no longer question why we have a shrine to Frida Kahlo in our house or wonder why our Christmas tree is decorated with queer icons and Albert Einstein. It no longer surprises me when you are bizarre, like the time you screech-stopped in the middle of a busy road because you thought you saw Stormzy in an off-licence. These days, I continue to shake my head at the way your mind works, secretly loving your weirdness.

But I was so angry with you for so long. The last few years, I was mad at everything, fuelled by rage, but somehow everything was related to you. It was misdirected, my anger, and I gave it all to you. I'm sorry for that. I'm sorry for a lot of things, and I know you are too. Even when we were far apart, or not communicating, you were always there, really, deep in my bones. I think that's what it means to have a mum.

Do you remember when I started primary school? I was so excited the first day. You waved me off at the gate, and I ran in, hardly turning around to wave back at you. But the second day, I couldn't understand why I was going back. I'd been already. Surely, that was it? Do you remember how I coiled around your leg, snake-like, and clung on, and you had to drag me in every day after that? I screamed so hard my face puffed out like a puffer fish. I didn't want to leave you. I didn't want to be apart from you. Even when you were annoying. Which was often.

Separating from you has always been the most painful thing. Maybe I had to make the last few years unbearable for both of us or I'd never be able to leave who you are and become completely myself. When you dropped me off at university, I could see the relief on your face. You'd been living in a hyper-anxious state worried that I might not even make it to eighteen. Without you I'd likely be dead. I'm glad to be alive. When it was time to say goodbye, you told me to 'walk fast, and don't look back'. But I'll always look back. And I know you'll always be there when I do.

You asked me a question when I stopped talking to you a few years ago that sums us up. We have always communicated, even if in strange ways. You sent a photo of your face as an apple, on a Snapchat filter, and the caption: How do you like them apples?

I like them apples a lot.

Ro X

A LETTER TO OUR READERS

Dear Readers,

We were unsure about writing this book. We wanted to speak out honestly and openly about what it means to be a teenager in this age, and what it means to parent one, but wondered who would want to read about our lives. After all, every single family and individual has their own story. We were also worried that in a few years we will probably have a totally different perspective on this time and change our minds about most things, because time does that. And of course, at certain times the idea of *working* together seemed ludicrous. But in the end, we decided to write *No Filters* as a no-holds-barred account of a moment in our lives. Because this is the book we both wish we had read.

Being a teenager is never, ever straightforward, but it seems that something catastrophic is going on at the moment and, wildly – it seems to us – our experience is not uncommon. Adolescent mental health issues are common, and desperately, desperately sad. There is much that we left out of *No Filters*, as it was too painful for both of us. Still, we were lucky. Too many young people do not have the support they urgently need. Although the storm has now passed, and we can laugh about most things, it is also acutely painful to remember some days, and maybe it will be like that always. It will take a long time to repair the scars from some of what Ro went through. Healing has begun. Our relationship is stronger than ever, but there are no quick-fixes to heal from mental illness or recover a fractious mother–daughter relationship.

We wanted to share our story in any case, in the hope that somebody who is reading it during the worst of times sees a glimmer of light at the end of a tunnel. The world is full of hate, but that we can have totally different perspectives and views yet can tolerate and even learn from each other gives us both hope. That Ro could come back from such a dark place, and smile and laugh again, seemed beyond impossible a mere few years ago.

Parenting a teenager with a mental health condition feels like being in the loneliest place in the world, that nobody who hasn't experienced it really understands. Being a mentally unwell teenager is even lonelier and so, so frightening. For a long time, we both felt unheard – and unseen – by each other and by everyone. But we were not alone. There are so many mothers and daughters – and father and sons and families – going through what we went through, right now, all over the country, and all over the world. This book is for them.

We see you.

Ro and Christie XX

Christie: *Sobbing.* I wish we'd had this book. I wish it had existed.

Rowan: *Sobbing.* Me too.

Christie: I hope it helps people.

Rowan: It will. I love you so much.

Christie: I love you more.

Glossary

Almond Mum/Mom

Typically, white suburban moms who were 90s girls and never accepted they had an eating disorder, so now they have to make it everyone else's problem. (Urban Dictionary)

Mob Wife

The 'mob wife' aesthetic can be achieved with bold accessories such as gold hoop earrings, a leopard print jacket or vintage fur – items that can often be found by shopping second-hand. (CNBC)

Pumpkin Spice

A shitty coffee flavour that all teenage to young thirty-something yuppie white chicks love. (Urban Dictionary)

Bossman

Bossman is a phrase used in London slang to define the man selling chicken and chips in the local chip shop around the corner. (Urban Dictionary)

Stick n Poke

A homemade tattoo for when you're under eighteen and can't find someone to illegally tatt you. It's basically just repeatedly stabbing yourself with a needle and ink. It eventually fades away. Somewhat popular among Gen Z. (Urban Dictionary)

Moon Water

Water that has been charged by the Moon. (*Cosmopolitan* magazine)

Neuro-spicy

Neuro-spicy is a term used by people who are neurodivergent (meaning people with ADHD, autism, and so on). It's simply just a silly little alternate term for a neurodivergent person to use and express themselves. (Urban Dictionary)

Coshed

To hit someone with a cosh. (Cambridge Dictionary)

Gym Girl Account

An Instagram/TikTok account of a Gym Girl – see also Fitness Model – a type of social media influencer who routinely provides unsolicited health, fitness, and wellness advice while actually having very little knowledge of kinesiology and physiology, or without having any relevant medical certification. The Fitness Model's grandiose sense of self allows them to think of themselves as a subject matter expert in all things gym, diet, and selfies. (Urban Dictionary)

ED Recovery Account

In these accounts, people share posts with raw depictions of the reality of eating disorder recovery: before-and-after images, pictures of food or of themselves with food, even hospital photos. (*The Washington Post*)

Karen

Middle-aged woman, typically blonde, who makes the solutions to others' problems an inconvenience to her although she isn't even remotely affected. (Urban Dictionary)

Becky

Becky is slang for a white woman who is happily ignorant and unaware of her whiteness but is complicit with the system that upholds her status. She is often overly dramatic when confronted about her whiteness. (NPR)

Resources

Podcasts

Changes with Annie Macmanus
Code Switch
Miss Me with Lily Allen and Miquita Oliver
Nice White Parents
Therapy for Black Girls
Therapy Works
Things Fell Apart by Jon Ronson
Young Again

Books

Judith Butler, *Who's Afraid of Gender*, 2024
Lorraine Candy, *'Mum, What's Wrong with You?': 101 Things Only Mothers of Teenage Girls Know*, 2021
Emma Dabiri, *Disobedient Bodies: Reclaim Your Unruly Beauty*, 2023
Reni Eddo-Lodge, *Why I'm No Longer Talking to White People About Race*, 2017
Natalie Evans and Naomi Evans, *The Mixed-Race Experience: Reflections and Revelations on Multiracial Identity*, 2022
Shon Faye, *The Transgender Issue: An Argument for Justice*, 2021
Bryony Gordon, *Mad Woman: How to Survive a World That Thinks You're the Problem*, 2024
Gabor Mate and Daniel Mate, *The Myth of Normal: Trauma, Illness, and Healing in a Toxic Culture*, 2022

Philippa Perry, *The Book You Wish Your Parents Had Read: (And Your Children Will Be Glad That You Did)*, 2019

Julie Phillips, *The Baby on the Fire Escape: Creativity, Motherhood and the Mind–Baby Problem*, 2022

Sylvia Plath, *The Bell Jar*, 1963

Robert Samuels and Toluse Olorunnipa, *His Name Is George Floyd: One Man's Life and the Struggle for Racial Justice*, 2022

Britt Wray, *Generation Dread: Finding Purpose in an Age of Eco-Anxiety*, 2022

Resources

BEAT, https://www.beateatingdisorders.org.uk/
Childline, https://www.childline.org.uk/
Samaritans, https://www.samaritans.org/
FRANK, https://www.talktofrank.com/
KOOTH, https://www.kooth.com/
Smartphone Free Childhood, https://smartphonefreechildhood.co.uk/
Young Minds, https://www.youngminds.org.uk/

Biographies

Christie is a writer and Professor of Medical Humanities at University of East Anglia. Rowan co-wrote this book between the ages of sixteen and eighteen, and is currently in her first year at university, studying Classics. They are both enjoying getting to know each other as adults, as mother and daughter, and as women.

Endnotes

Chapter Two

1 John Harris, 'The Mother of Neurodiversity: How Judy Singer Changed the World', *The Guardian*, 5 July 2023, available at https://www.theguardian.com/world/2023/jul/05/the-mother-of-neurodiversity-how-judy-singer-changed-the-world.
2 See https://www.bbk.ac.uk/research/centres/neurodiversity-at-work.
3 Rachel Williams, 'Wired Differently: How Neurodiversity Adds New Skillsets to the Workforce', *The Guardian*, 25 August 2023, available at https://www.theguardian.com/global-development/2023/aug/25/wired-differently-how-neurodiversity-adds-new-skillsets-to-the-workplace.
4 Darby E. Attoe and Emma A. Climie, 'Miss Diagnosis – A Systemic Review of ADHD in Adult Women', *J Atten Disord*, 27(7), May 2023: 645–657.
5 National Autistic Society, 'Autistic Women and Girls', available at https://www.autism.org.uk/advice-and-guidance/what-is-autism/autistic-women-and-girls.

Chapter Three

6 WWD (Women's Wear Daily), 'Kate Moss: The Waif That Roared', 13 November 2009, available at https://wwd.com/feature/kate-moss-the-waif-that-roared-2367932-1410207/.
7 Children's Commissioner, 'Young People with Eating Disorders

in England on the Rise', 1 August 2023, available at https://www.childrenscommissioner.gov.uk/blog/young-people-with-eating-disorders-in-england-on-the-rise/.

8 *The Guardian*, 'UK Eating Disorder Charity Says Calls from People with Arfid Have Risen Sevenfold', 27 February 2024, available at https://www.theguardian.com/society/2024/feb/26/uk-eating-disorder-arfid-avoidant-restrictive-food-intake-disorder-nhs.

9 NHS England, 'One in Five Children and Young People Had a Probable Mental Disorder in 2023', 21 November 2023, available at https://www.england.nhs.uk/2023/11/one-in-five-children-and-young-people-had-a-probable-mental-disorder-in-2023/.

10 National Institute for Health and Care Excellence, 'Eating Disorders: How Common is it?', revised July 2019, available at https://cks.nice.org.uk/topics/eating-disorders/background-information/prevalence/.

Chapter Five

11 'Social Media Could Be as Harmful to Children as Smoking or Gambling – Why Is This Allowed?', *The Guardian*, 4 July 2023, available at https://www.theguardian.com/commentisfree/2023/jul/04/smoking-gambling-children-social-media-apps-snapchat-health-regulation.

12 Alice Park, 'The U.S. Surgeon General Fears Social Media Is Harming the "Well-Being of Our Children"', *Time*, 23 May 2023, availableathttps://time.com/6282893/surgeon-general-vivek-murthy-interview-social-media/.

13 Jean Twenge, 'Teenage Depression and Suicide Are Way Up – and So Is Smartphone Use', *The Washington Post*, 19 November 2017, available at https://www.washingtonpost.com/national/health-science/teenage-depression-and-suicide-are-way-up-and-so-is-smartphone-use/2017/11/17/624641ea-ca13-11e7-8321-481fd63f174d_story.html; Priory, 'Should Children Have Smartphones?',

22 August 2018, available at https://www.priorygroup.com/blog/should-children-really-have-their-own-smartphones.

Chapter Six

14 *The Guardian*, ' "If You Ask Me, I Am British": Joys and Trials for Britain's Multi-Ethnic Households', 2 December 2022, available at https://www.theguardian.com/uk-news/2022/dec/02/joys-trials-britains-increasingly-mixed-race-households-census-2021.

15 Aaliyah Miller, 'Mixed Women Explain Why Talking about Race with Their Families Matters', Refinery29, 29 March 2021, availableathttps://www.refinery29.com/en-gb/racism-in-mixed-race-families.

16 Nissa Finney, James Nazroo, Laia Bécares, Dharmi Kapadia, and Natalie Shlomo, eds, 'Racism and Ethnic Inequality in a Time of Crisis: Findings from the Evidence for Equality National Survey', 12 April 2023, available at https://bristoluniversitypressdigital.com/edcollbook-oa/book/9781447368861/9781447368861.xml.

17 Nadine White, 'Just 1% of UK Professors Are Black, New Figures Reveal', *Independent*, February 2022, available at https://www.independent.co.uk/news/uk/home-news/uk-professors-black-government-figures-b2004891.html.

Chapter Seven

18 Melody Schreiber, 'Addressing Climate Change Concerns in Practice', *Monitor on Psychology*, 52(2), 1 March 2021, available at https://www.apa.org/monitor/2021/03/ce-climate-change.

19 Matt McGrath, 'Climate Change: Polar Bears Face Starvation Threat as Ice Melts', BBC, 13 February 2024, available at https://www.bbc.com/news/science-environment-68253819.

20 Mark Poynting, 'World's First Year-Long Breach of Key 1.5C

Warming Limit', BBC, available at https://www.bbc.co.uk/news/science-environment-68110310#:~:text=For%20the%20first%20time%2C%20global,avoid%20the%20most%20damaging%20impacts.

21 Aliya Uteuova, 'Nearly 15% of Americans Don't Believe Climate Change Is Real, Study Finds', *The Guardian*, 14 February 2024, available at https://www.theguardian.com/us-news/2024/feb/14/americans-believe-climate-change-study#:~:text=The%20findings%20are%20consistent%20with,(about%2049%20million%20people).

22 Fiona Cowood, ' "You Feel Like a Failure": The Parents Driven to Despair by Their Children's Refusal to Go to School, *The Telegraph*, 3 February 2024, available at https://www.telegraph.co.uk/news/2024/02/03/ghost-children-school-absence-refusal-parents-mental-health/.

23 Caroline Hickman et al., 'Climate Anxiety in Children and Young People and Their Beliefs about Government Responses to Climate Change: A Global Survey', *The Lancet*, December 2021, available at https://www.thelancet.com/journals/lanplh/article/PIIS2542-5196(21)00278-3/fulltext.